July 2015

Dear Margie,

Thanks for your friendship, and leadership of all things good in healthcare!

Paul U.

OAK PRAIRIE
HEALTH PRESS

Field Guide to Collaborative Care

Implementing the Future of Health Care

Paul Uhlig and W. Ellen Raboin

ISBN 978-0-9914112-9-0

Oak Prairie Health Press | Overland Park, Kansas USA

This is the highest compliment:
"You treated us like ordinary people,
and that made all the difference."

CONTENTS

4 ACTIVATING

5 DEEPENING

6 SUSTAINING

7 SOCIAL FIELD MODEL

INTRODUCTION

The work described in the *Field Guide to Collaborative Care* started with a question. More precisely, it began when a care team decided to make a painful and puzzling question go away. That question, asked too often by patients and family members, is "Don't you people talk to each other?"

Of course people in health care talk to each other. They talk, text, call, write orders and notes, and spend long days and nights trying their best to care for their patients. Entire information platforms are devoted to this. Yet despite hard work and careful attention, traditional health care often leaves patients and families feeling confused and alienated instead of secure; leaves health care professionals feeling frustrated and discouraged instead of fulfilled; and produces care that can be unsafe, with quality that can be surprisingly poor and uneven, and costs that are out of control. How can this be?

"Don't you people talk to each other?" Yes...but... Why doesn't it feel like they do, and why aren't care outcomes better?

Why aren't health care professionals, patients, and family members – all working with good intent – able to produce the kind of care that everyone intends and expects? The explanation isn't about the abilities of people working in health care or their dedication, nor is it about technology, and certainly it isn't about the hopes, desires, and commitment of patients and families. The answer is in the way that care happens. A different way of working together is needed that produces better results.

This book is about understanding and implementing a promising new future for health care. Together with patients and families, we and our colleagues have experienced a better way of working in health care that makes this question go away – it is called collaborative care. The future of health care is achievable today. It is much better! Come see!

We feel on many days as if we and our colleagues are explorers pressing forward with wonder and excitement into a fascinating new frontier. This book is our report back to you – and an invitation to join in this meaningful work.

We begin by considering distinctions between collaborative care and traditional care, first in stories and then with observations. In additional sections we offer reflections and specific recommendations about how collaborative care can be successfully implemented – how to prepare, and how to activate, deepen, and sustain your work. Throughout the Field Guide we provide detailed descriptions of approaches and actions that we have found to be helpful from firsthand experience.

The Field Guide to Collaborative Care is based on a conceptual framework known as the *Social Field Model of Collaborative Care.* The model was developed as a way of understanding collaborative care and how it can be intentionally implemented, and for facilitating the emergence of reliability and resilience with active patient and family engagement.

We hope that you will find the *Field Guide to Collaborative Care* interesting and useful, and that you will consider adding to it by contributing your own experiences and insights on the Collaborative Care Alliance website at www.cca-home.org by becoming part of the Collaborative Care Learning Network.

We welcome talking with you! Join us!

Paul Uhlig, MD
Wichita, Kansas

Ellen Raboin, PhD
Danville, California

INVITATION

Come with us...

We are in a patient care room. Look around: This room has been built for a purpose. Here is a bed. Here is a seating area. Here is a window. Here is a monitor. Here is a place for supplies. Here is a computer. Everything is clean, in place, and ready.

What has happened here before? Who has been cared for in this room? What joys and sorrows have been shared here? What will happen here tomorrow?

Sometime later today or tomorrow this room will come to life. Lights will be turned on, the monitor will be connected, a patient will rest in the bed, and family members will sit in the chairs or make cell phone calls by the window.

Nurses will be present and doctors will come. Throughout the day and night many health care professionals will care for the patient, talk with the patient and family, enter notes in the record, communicate with one another, and carry out their work together.

As these things are happening, hover over the care environment and see what you notice:

- Do people here seem to know just what to expect of each other and what to do together?
- Are people here alert, responsive, respectful, and patient with each other?
- Does everyone seem to feel invited and welcomed here, sharing ideas and suggestions?

- Do you see intentional and receptive engagement with patients and families?
- Do you see a seamless web of monitoring so that anything unexpected is quickly recognized?
- Is there a noticeable commitment to learning and change among everyone here?
- Are ideas and suggestions emerging that don't seem to come from any one person?
- Is there a sense of aliveness of the human spirit that makes care here unusually meaningful?

If you can answer a clear "yes" to all of these questions, you are experiencing a rich, vibrant social field in which the special contextual resources of collaborative care are flourishing. If you cannot answer "yes" to these questions, you are experiencing a less capable social field in which these resources are not yet well developed.

In the same way that physical environments can be intentionally designed and built, social environments for exceptional care can be intentionally and purposefully created. The *Field Guide to Collaborative Care* is a blueprint for doing that.

Something new is about to happen! Come with us!

Photo:
Collaborative Care Team
Wesley Medical Center
Wichita, Kansas

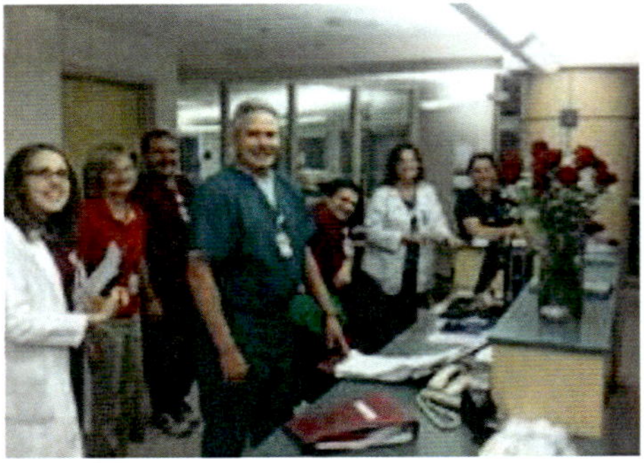

PROLOGUE

Mary's story

Mary (daughter, maternal-child nurse, nursing educator):

My mother's name was Nina. She was an 82-year-old independent woman. Her parents were German Mennonites. She had 16 brothers and sisters. Growing up she spoke English, but she also spoke Low German at home. When she first woke up after the accident she spoke in that Low German. My husband can speak a little, so he talked with her and she talked right back.

She finished 8th grade. Further education was not encouraged. She was a homemaker. She cleaned for a living – into her 80s. She said, "I need things to do." She and my father were completely active, completely cognizant. She worked right up to before the accident, cleaning a doctor's office.

She was an excellent cook. She liked to bake. She was not outgoing, but she spent a lot of time with her grandchildren. Her grandchildren made her laugh. They brought her joy. She had a special thing about our son. When he was little she referred to him as "my boy." When my son came to visit her in the hospital she said, "That's my boy!"

It was December – it's been thirteen years already. My parents were going out to dinner with another couple. Another driver crossed the center line and there was a head-on accident. The two friends were killed at the scene. My mother was thrown out of the car and critically injured, a head injury. My father, who was the least healthy, was the least injured.

He was taken to a smaller hospital near where they lived. My mother was airlifted to the larger medical center here. Their pastor called me. I tracked her down.

At first when I got to the hospital they wouldn't let me be with her because they had not identified her. I am her daughter and a nurse. I was standing right there telling them she was my mother. After a phone call to the sheriff, they finally let me in.

Her care in the ICU was fine. Everything seemed very well organized. They let me come in anytime. The first move was to a step down floor. She sort of stabilized and started waking up.

Because of her head injury, she couldn't swallow well. The speech therapist seeing her was very good. She wrote out very clear instructions that she taped over the bed: NOT TO BE LEFT ALONE WHEN SHE EATS. But often they would just bring her tray in and walk out. When I asked, her nurse would say, "She fed herself just fine. Everything was great." I knew it couldn't be fine, because I helped her eat and she couldn't do it.

Her accident was on December 5th, and she died on January 7th. In those 33 days she was moved five times. Every time she moved, a piece of her history was lost. By the time she died back in a different ICU they didn't even know she had been in a car accident or had a head injury. They thought she was a nursing home patient.

Christmas Day was the worst. Her feeding tube was sliding in and out where it hadn't healed well and had a lot of irritation around it. My mother just kept wanting to scratch the area. I spent most of the day holding her hands. My daughter came and helped care for her so I could spend a little time with the rest of our family. When I got back, she said, "Mom, all I've done is just hold her."

A new tube was ordered, but there were things they needed from other places and the pharmacy. This went on the entire day. Finally, around 9 p.m., another physician showed up. She was part of the trauma team, but I'd never met her. She said,

"We can do better than this." But she said we would have to wait for the supplies. And then she looked around the room and the supplies were right there. They had been there the whole time.

While the doctor was there, they brought a sandwich for my mother. There was no way she could swallow that. The nursing assistant grabbed the sandwich and held it out to the doctor. She said, "Her daughter says she can't eat this. What diet order do you want?" This is where I found that I was the one reporting what was going on. If I didn't do it, it would be forgotten.

They didn't talk to each other. A resident or whoever would come in, and I would tell that person what had happened. The speech therapist provided good care, and I am sure she wrote in the chart about the changes she was seeing, but I don't think anyone else knew about it.

Her mental status was changing, and she wasn't eating. I really found that shift-to-shift, nurse to nurse, there were big pieces of things missed. There were things they didn't know. They didn't get it unless they got it from me. As a family member, you have to ask and do it because no one else will.

Another resident showed up and was worried about her calories, but the intake wasn't being recorded and no one really knew how much she was actually eating. What they also didn't know was that everything she ate was leaking out around her feeding tube. Food was leaking out around her tube, but nobody even knew that.

The case manager came in one day. She said, "Hasn't the team talked with you about what they decided at the team meeting?" I was furious. What team meeting? When they told me about the team meeting, it made me angry. How dare you have a meeting without including me, when I'm here 12 hours a day?

I wanted so badly for the cardiologist, trauma surgeon, and speech therapist to be all together in the room at the same time. I really don't know if the cardiologist knew what else was going on with her. Would he have made a different decision about the Coumadin if they had done that? My wish was: Get them together.

My father spent a lot of time with her. My niece brought him up there, 50 miles every day. During that time he was pretty much ignored. He was an elderly man in a wheelchair.

And – they all knew I was a nurse. As soon as someone found out I was a nurse, they quit talking to my dad. They would just talk to me. And the language would go up a notch. I would just know that was going to happen. So – don't forget who is in the room. If the husband of the patient is in the room, don't ignore him, even if he is in a wheelchair.

Her cognition continued to decrease. On a Saturday her nurse was concerned. The pastor was in and wanted to know if he should say a prayer. So we gathered by the bed and while we were standing there I heard this popping sound. There was bright red blood on the sheet. The nurse called the resident and they moved her to the ICU. They hung one bag of blood after another.

The next morning her main physician came. That was the first time he had introduced himself to my father after all that time. He said, "Things are not looking really good." Well, of course things were not looking really good. We knew that.

I was so tired. That afternoon a lot of family and friends showed up, and my brother arrived from Oregon. I was heading for the elevator to get some rest when they called me back. She had stopped breathing. They started to code her, but my brother went in and stopped it, and she died. Thank goodness he had the presence of mind to do that. A resident pronounced her dead. We never saw any of the staff or physicians from the trauma team.

When it was all over, I was sad for my dad because it shouldn't have happened that way. I was angry for a long time, and sad. It was all I could think about. I don't think any errors were committed on purpose – but they never talked to each other. I keep wondering, if they had talked to each other, would things have turned out differently? And I am crying, so I have to stop. It is 13 years later and I am still crying.

I was out for a walk several years ago and ran into a man I know. He had been the band teacher for our children. He needed to talk. So we stood on the street corner and I listened. His wife was ill, in the hospital. He told the same story – they don't talk to each other. I said – ask for a social worker. I gave him some suggestions of what to ask for. Later, he called me. Things were going poorly. A few days later she died. I went over to his home. He just spent the evening talking about her, showing me her quilts. He kept telling me the same story, what went on.

If I say anything about this to people, I immediately get another story from whoever I am talking to. There are lots of these stories out there. People say, "Well, you know, this one says this, and that one says that, and I don't know what to think anymore."

My wish? That whoever reads this can see there is a better way. There is no intention to give poor care, but it happens. We can do better.

As a nursing educator, I know this has informed what I do. It is why I am so passionate about interprofessional education. Just communicating across professions would make such a difference. That is always in my head – we can do better.

Clarence's story

Janette (daughter):

It felt like we became a family. I tell you what, we just came back for the first time and everyone here has greeted us. It's like we've come back home again.

I'm a three-time cancer survivor. I think this one just felt like we were really part of Dad's team. I really appreciated people listening to things I noticed about him and respecting what I said.

I asked my sister what she thought, because she knew I would be talking with you. She said to tell you that it was an honor being treated as a human – that we had an input to Dad's care.

The nursing staff was so humble. They treated us like one of their own. We felt respected. I guess you could sum it up by saying, "It was a good experience in a bad situation." That isn't what we would have expected.

At the beginning of rounds each day, each person was asked for their input. We felt included as a family. We felt we had the right to say something. It was also interesting how the nurses responded to it. They were very respectful, and they included us.

We had one incident that was a shocker for us with a nurse who was new to Dad's nursing staff. She did not treat us with the same kind of respect we had become used to. It was very difficult. We realized what a difference it had made for us.

Ilene (wife):

I don't know the words, but we felt accepted to be in that circle every morning. It was a team. We got to learn what each one was doing and thinking. It was so informative.

If someone said something should change, people would listen and say maybe let's do that. I never expected a hospital stay to be like that. We wouldn't miss those 8:30 meetings for anything.

Janette:

For me, I was learning what meds Dad was on, what his condition really was. We were privileged to the medical part of his care. I took a lot of notes every day, and I've used them with other doctors since leaving the hospital to find out what his medical condition really is.

One thing we liked was the goal board. One of the nurses would write on it, and sometimes my sister did that on rounds. It was a good checklist to be sure nothing got missed. The next day somebody would read it. We put some simple things on it: shower, hair combed, shaved. These things were very important to him.

I've told people that our experiences were such a neat experience. We were there for such an awful situation, but we looked forward to being on that floor every day.

Clarence (patient):

The other times I've been in the hospital, a lot of the time I felt like I'm a monkey in the zoo. Here I felt like part of a family. It really was. When I was recovering I felt like I was a baby. I had to learn everything over again. It added a lot to my healing to know that all of these people cared.

Janette:

Many times we hold doctors or people above us. We don't think we can relate to them. Here, it wasn't like that.

Finding even better ways

Health care is evolving.

Time-honored ways of working in health care are no longer meeting the needs of patients, families, and society. Nor are they meeting the personal and professional hopes and needs of the health care workforce.

The paradox of present day health care is that – on the one hand – health care professionals are among the most highly motivated, highly trained in any area of human endeavor. Health care professionals prepare for years, work as hard and as well as possible, and are deeply dedicated to the care of their patients.

Yet – on the other hand – health care faces major unsolved challenges that are progressing. Health care costs are increasing at unsustainable rates. Quality and safety are surprisingly uneven and not what we wish they would be. Limitations to access affect almost every sector of society from individuals to families to businesses to nations. And the experiences of giving or receiving care – which should be one of the most rewarding of human exchanges – often feel depressing and discouraging instead of renewing and fulfilling.

What is also interesting is that the growing and unsolved challenges of *cost, quality, access, and experience of care* are not unique to this country. They are global – manifesting in every country across the world where health care is approached, organized and practiced in modern traditional ways.

How can this be?

Health care presently exists between paradigms. The old ways in which health care has been organized and practiced for over a century are no longer working, yet the new ways that are needed haven't been fully developed or possibly even imagined. This is a time in health care that is uncomfortable, stressful, and uncertain – and yet...filled with potential.

Futurist Ian Morrison and quality expert Martin Merry talk about two curves of health care. The first curve represents health care's current paradigm. Although the first curve has hundreds of years of antecedents, it has a birthdate, 1893, when the Johns Hopkins Medical School was founded. In the pioneering work of the founding faculty at Johns Hopkins, including William Osler and others, present ways of organizing, working, and teaching in medicine were brought together for the first time. The first curve has a second major milestone, 1910, when the Flexner report about the state of medical education across the US was published. That report offered a new model, the Hopkins model.

In other health professions, including nursing beginning with the pioneering work of Florence Nightingale, similar transformations were happening. The world was ready for this inspired revolution, and within decades a dramatic transformation occurred in how health care was organized, practiced and taught across the US and across the world. The result was the birth of our present paradigm in health care. For most of the last century, these ways of organizing, practicing and teaching health care brought remarkable benefits.

As with all human progress, health care has continued to evolve and change. Incrementally at first, and then with progressive force and significance, innovations in health care that once were revolutionary no longer serve health care well. Understandings and insights and needs have grown beyond them.

Just like a century ago, traditional ways of working in health care are poised for transformation. Those of us working in health care share with society the privilege of participating in a once-in-a-hundred-year moment: the birth of a new paradigm.

We illustrate the old and the emerging new paradigms of health care below with two curves. The second curve is drawn with a dashed line, because it represents deep innovations of a new future of health care that cannot be fully known or imagined yet from our present understandings.

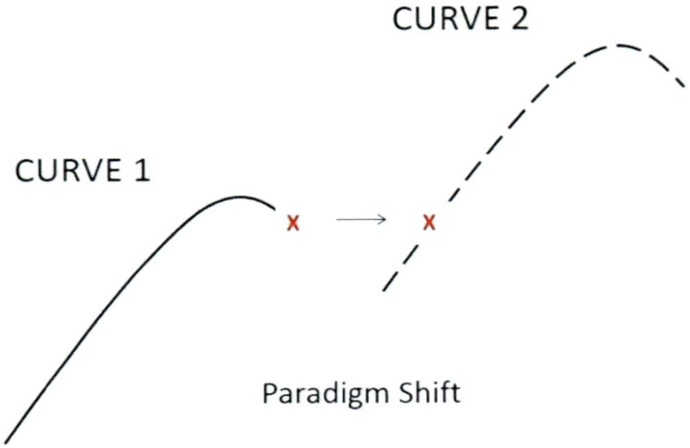

Figure: A Once-in-a-Hundred Year Moment -
Curve One and Curve Two Health Care (Merry/Morrison)

As active participants in the creation of the Second Curve, we believe that how health care feels for practitioners depends on which curve you are on. For many people this is a sad and difficult time in health care. No wonder. For a person deeply immersed in Curve One health care, everything that person knows and has dedicated his or her life to, is no longer working. For a Curve One practitioner or institution, the present era in health care can be a time of profound frustration and loss, a time of mourning the inexorable disappearance of something dear and treasured.

However, an increasing number of people have done that grieving and moved beyond it. Together with patients, family members and society at large, they are actively participating in the thrilling task of helping to create the new world of health care.

Instead of resisting or mourning the death of Curve One, they are engaged in the fascinating birth of Curve Two. When you visit these people and their institutions, your skin will practically tingle with the excitement they feel about the work they are doing – filled with meaning, aliveness and hope.

Although it is not possible to know yet exactly what form Curve Two health care will eventually take, it is clear that efforts to implement and understand collaborative care and to actively engage patients and family members in care are important steps. These actions create the conditions from which insights and experiences leading to Curve Two can emerge.

So, how do we do this?

Let's imagine that we are members of a care team interested in transforming our practice together. We have a vision of taking intentional steps toward Second Curve health care. We read the literature for ideas and guidance – "collaborative care," "high reliability teamwork with engagement of patients and families" – these sound exciting and worthwhile. We, too, want to do an even better job caring for our patients. "Let's try," one of us says. "Sounds good." "Let's do it." But… What, exactly, should we do? Here are some possibilities we might consider.

A lot has been written about high reliability and resilience. Maybe we should study and teach those principles to our team as a way of bringing those approaches into our daily practice. So we read the literature, talk with experts in teamwork, and get leadership support. Some of us go away for TeamSTEPPS™

training. Those people have a great time together and return full of excitement. A train-the-trainer program is established, and multidisciplinary rounds is started. Some people like the changes, but others don't. Some people are interested, yet others hold back or push back. Many people seem passive or even hostile. People say their ordinary work takes longer and seems harder rather than better or safer. We are puzzled. We watch the data: A few things improve, but overall people are not happier and most outcomes do not change. Why?

"Actually," one of us says, "all we really need are better protocols." "Look what the literature shows when this protocol was used for glycemic control, when this one was used for sepsis, when this one was used for line insertions, and when this one was used for elective C-sections." So we call our practitioners to a meeting and show them the protocols, intending to implement them here. In certain areas we are successful. In others, the resistance is strong and we can't get there. When we look at the data we are puzzled. Some of the units using the new protocols aren't any better, and some of the units that resisted adopting the new protocols have the best outcomes. Why?

Maybe we should try a different method. The CEO says, "Work with a six sigma black belt and start a Lean initiative." The consultant brings people together, maps processes, and looks for waste to eliminate and things to standardize. Run charts go up on the wall. We have tables colored red, yellow, and green: Core Measures, Patient Satisfaction, Top Box scores. We hire additional people to manage data and let us know when doctors, units or managers don't perform. We create incentives, some positive, some punitive. A few measures do shift. Others don't. Sometimes breakthroughs happen. More often, changes are small and don't last. Why?

Right now our energy is really low. We are overwhelmed. Our new computer order entry system is taking every moment of our attention. We are training staff and physicians night and day, trying to meet the "Go Live!" deadline. Our new system crashes. Order sets are lost. Pieces of paper go on the wall: "Only select 'Reconcile Meds' on discharge!!" Plenty of breakfasts and special meetings later, people are mostly able to get their work done with only an hour or so of extra effort every day. The temporary IT staff is gradually getting smaller. We look at the data: Length of stay is the same, work takes more time, practitioners aren't happy, and most medication errors haven't changed. Why?

Maybe what we need is to get our "Board on Board," and begin leadership safety rounds. So we try these: a quality and safety board committee is formed, and leadership safety rounds are made every week. New connections are formed and awareness is heightened. An overwhelming stream of safety concerns comes from the safety rounds, almost too many to cope with. It is hard to follow up and close the loop back to the front line staff. The Director of Quality is held accountable and replaced. Some measures improve and are celebrated. Our CEO gives a presentation at a national safety meeting. Yet people on the front line remain skeptical and "never events" continue to happen. Safety attitude survey results improve on several units but on most don't change. Safety rounds is pushed to monthly. Why?

Or maybe, we are amazingly successful! Then, just as our collaborative care initiative is really getting good, reality sets in. Our energized front line collaborative care team with participatory leadership and emergent capabilities turns out to be a poor fit in the traditional leadership structure of our health care organization. Our collaborative care initiative, even with notable and measurable successes and honors, is tolerated for a while but increasingly is perceived as needing to be more aligned with the policies, procedures, and management methods that our health care organization relies on and believes are required. Eventually these organizational processes – well intended and designed to do what our collaborative care team does by its very nature as easily as breathing – arise with bureaucratic ferocity to put the errant wild child to rest. Why? And, we keep hearing from providers, "I wish I had more time to really care for my patients!" and from patients and family members, "Don't you people talk to each other?"

A new future waiting

If these stories and comments sound familiar, you are actively engaged at the cutting edge of health care practice and leadership, wherever modern scientific health care practice is the norm across the US and the world. You are participating in well-intended efforts to transform care with a purpose of improving quality, lowering costs, making health care more accessible, and increasing satisfaction.

Yet, despite years of scholarship and effort, there remain many more unsolved puzzles than insights and successes. The future of health care is a wide open frontier.

This guide is written by peers who are traveling the same journey as you. The changes needed in health care are profound. With each step forward it is possible to see farther into an exciting new future for health care. We have come far enough now to realize that the very foundations of health care are changing – MUST change for the degree of transformation that is required.

The future of health care requires more than doing what we have always done, only in better or more efficient ways. Our fundamental approaches, our professional identities, what we teach our children, and even our purposes must evolve and change. It will happen, and it is happening now.

The *Field Guide to Collaborative Care* presents a new way of thinking about the changes needed in health care, with fresh insights about how to achieve them. It is a journal of experiences and lessons learned, an early roadmap for this transformational journey, from a new perspective.

The past and present of health care are well known from our ordinary experiences, whether as patients and family members, or as health care professionals. A new future of health care is waiting to be written. It will come into being through the collective imagination, hard work, thoughtful decisions, courage, hopes, insights, and new beliefs of care teams, patients and family members across the world – co-created moment by moment through pioneering explorations and innovations.

This is an interesting time in health care. If you are an established practitioner, many things aren't working like they used to, and the future is very uncertain. If you are a student, you must still learn the old ways of doing things to a level of mastery. For all of us – seasoned or beginning – our most important professional work concerns envisioning and building the new paradigm.

The privilege of creating a new paradigm falls only to a handful of generations at pivotal moments in history. For more than a hundred years, people in health care have known only the old paradigm. For no reason other than we are all here, on duty as these changes are taking place, it falls to us to create the new future of health care. This is a once-in-a hundred-year moment. Change is happening here, now. It is exciting and rewarding.

You can be part of this fascinating work! Join us!

PART ONE

RECOGNIZING COLLABORATIVE CARE

- Distinctions between Traditional and Collaborative Care
- A View of Traditional Multidisciplinary Rounds
- A View of Collaborative Care
- A Turning Point

Distinctions between Traditional and Collaborative Care

We have a very ambitious definition of collaborative care. We define collaborative care as exceptional health care in which patients, family members, and other care team members are able to consistently *co-create care that is meaningful, safe, reliable, resilient, efficient, and exquisitely responsive to the hopes, needs, goals, and purposes of everyone involved*. In our experience this definition is achievable.

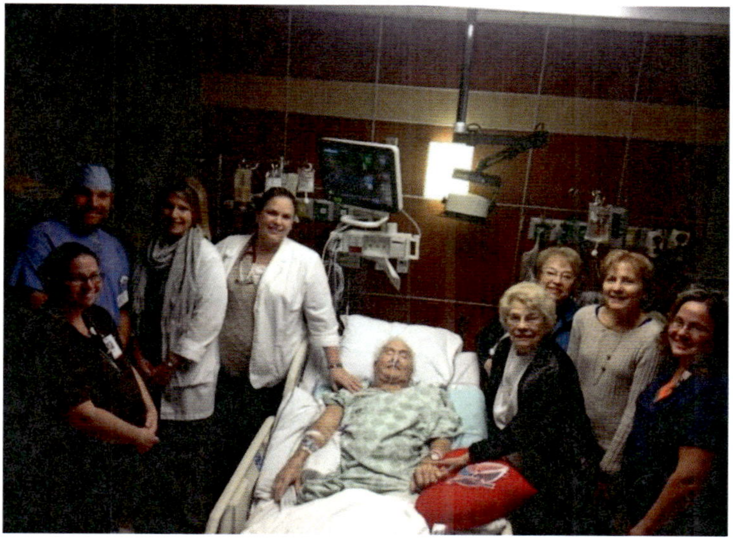

Figure: Collaborative Care, Salina Regional Health Center, Salina, Kansas

The core elements of collaborative care are: 1) active engagement of patients and families in all aspects of care and decision making, 2) exceptional teamwork across the entire interprofessional team, and 3) ongoing team learning and system monitoring and improvement to achieve reliability and resilience.

In this section we will consider what collaborative care looks like and how you can know it when you see it. However, the even more interesting question is how to make collaborative care happen. Our research points to many underlying factors in the care environment that are important for collaborative care to happen well. Collaborative care is much more than what takes place at the bedside.The threads of collaborative care are woven across every part of the entire care enviornment.

Throughout this book we will discuss the breadth of these differences in structure, staffing, learning, and leadership. This book is about the "How" of collaborative care as much or more than the "What." However, as a beginning, in this introduction we highlight observable differences between traditional health care practice and collaborative care – focusing on how collaborative care team members work together, and how patients and families are included as active participants in care activities.

Observable differences

In our research we often observe care teams doing their work. As we observe care, we watch for who is included in care activities, and how each role and person is integrated or not in daily work routines. The roles we observe include patients, families, physicians, nurse practitioners, physician assistants, nurses, pharmacists, respiratory therapists, physical therapists and physical therapy assistants, care coordinators, social workers, chaplains, nutritionists, residents, medical students, nursing students, and other care providers such as patient care assistants.

Imagine being with a care team as they care for a patient. Envision what people are doing, and observe the following things:

Where does care happen? Who is present? What happens before an episode of care? How do people enter the patient's room? Do people sit at eye level, or stand? If present, are family members included in the bedside group? How do the conversations begin? Who leads? Who does most of the talking? What are people paying attention to? Can you tell right away about the patient as a person? Is the language used medical or ordinary? Do people report about the patient saying "he" or "she," or do people talk with the patient and family saying "you"? What does the hierarchy feel like? Do people feel comfortable speaking up? As a routine part of care, does anyone ask if anything could have gone better? Are mistakes and errors openly discussed? Is a safety checklist used? Is the care plan written down, summarized, and clearly understood by everyone present? Are professional care team members, patients, and family members clearly engaged in doing something together that has meaning for them?

We are looking for more than presence. It is one thing for different health professionals, patients, and family members to be present together in a care environment, and another for these people to be actively participating together in meaningful ways.

A View of Traditional Multidisciplinary Rounds

When we ask about collaborative care, people often say, "We do that already." However, when we observe care teams in a traditional care environment, this is what we usually see:

Professional care team members frequently meet in a conference room or talk in the hallway outside of the patient's room before going in to see the patient. In teaching environments, the attending physician, residents, and medical students often meet separately from nurses and other professional team members. These interactions before entering the patient's room usually happen without involvement of the patient and family.

Important discussions occur and significant decisions are made in these "pre-meetings."

Once entering the patient's room, people move directly to reports about what has happened. Only rarely does the process begin with introductions, or with invitations to participate. Although many health professionals and students may be present, only a few people do most of the talking. There is a definite sense of hierarchy. Physicians usually lead the process while other professionals are asked or directed to report about their area of expertise. The format includes reports about the patient, questions and answers, and instructions. The pace is frequently brisk.

When people speak, they usually direct their attention to the physician or to other members of the care team, reporting about the patient in the third person as "he" or "she" rather than looking at and talking with the patient and family. The patient is usually not an active participant in most of the discussions that take place. Although the process is almost always professional and respectful, the content, tone, and flow of the conversations happen in ways that are not conducive to patient inclusion. Instead the patient is told, listens, and answers specific questions.

Family members are rarely active participants. In fact, families are not usually with the patients. Visiting hour restrictions or timing of rounds often prevent families from being present when plans are being made. Communicating with the family is considered something to be done later in the day.

The focus of the conversations is mostly about medical details of the patient's condition and communicating a plan of care. It is hard to know about the patient as a person from what is talked about. The language used has many technical terms that are hard for non-professionals to understand. Patients and family members are told what is happening rather than being invited to participate in developing an understanding of the patient's condition and jointly developing a plan of care.

Certain parts of the conversation apply to certain people, but other parts don't. At times, care team professionals look at papers or computers, check messages, leave the room, accomplish tasks, and have whispered side conversations when others are talking.

Errors or mistakes are not discussed if patients and family members are present. System concerns are not asked about. A safety checklist is not usually used. Rarely is a closing summary discussed or a review of plans and responsibilities. The main decisions from rounds are documented in the patient's chart; however, usually no record is left behind for the patient or family.

A View of Collaborative Care

In contrast, when we observe care teams in highly evolved collaborative care environments, this is what we see:

Patients and family members are invited and encouraged to participate in rounds and all other care activities. Family members can be with patients at any time of the day or night, and are told in advance that the care team will come at a specific time and that they are invited to participate.

Care conversations before going into the patient's room are minimized. Professional care team members intentionally wait until they are present with the patient and family members before having any conversations about how the patient is doing and before any plans for care are made.

Members of the care team visibly wash or foam their hands as they enter the patient's room. They gather around the patient, inviting and welcoming family members to join with them in their circle. People often sit at eye level with the patient.

The care conversation begins with introductions of everyone present, including health care professionals, the patient, and family members, with invitations to join and participate. Time is taken to ask and learn about the interests of patient and family as people, and to establish connections among everyone participating. The tone is respectful, relaxed, and inviting.

There is a clear pattern and sequence that professional care team members are familiar with and that patients and families soon learn and join. The care conversation is led by various people at different times, depending on what is being discussed. Often a nurse practitioner or other care team member, other than a physician, facilitates and guides the process.

Physicians are active participants in the conversations and decision making but do not always lead or direct. Deference is given and leadership flows based on the expertise needed at the moment among all people present, including the expertise of the patient and family members, rather than professional hierarchy.

Interactions among people feel like a conversation rather than a report. A shared understanding of what is happening emerges in real time as people talk together. Plans are jointly developed as care team members, patients, and family members contribute various perspectives and discuss these with each other.

Everyone present is clearly engaged in a cohesive group conversation. There are few side conversations. People talk comfortably with each other and with the patient and family using "you" instead of "he" or "she." The language is ordinary rather than technical, and when technical and professional terms and concepts are used, they are immediately explained. Laughter happens frequently, often with joking or teasing. The tone is respectful, warm, and human.

Everyone is given an opportunity to contribute around the circle in turn, including patients and family members. Ideas flow among the assembled team, often without anyone directing or guiding the flow of the conversation. Frequently, new ideas emerge that were sparked by these interactions.

A safety checklist is used to be sure that essential items have been reviewed and discussed. Time is taken to ask if anything could have happened differently or better over the past 24 hours. Any mistakes or errors are openly discussed. Any problems or concerns are noted and documented for later review in a weekly system meeting.

The plan of care created during the conversation is written down on a goal board as it is developed. Any ambiguities and contingency plans are clarified. The goal board is reviewed and responsibilities clarified as a closing action. The goal board is left in the room as a reminder for anyone, including patients and family members, to see or review later, for example at shift-to-shift handovers. The care conversation the next day includes a point-by-point review of the plan on the goal board.

When the conversation ends, it is apparent that everyone in the room has a clear understanding of how the patient is doing and what the plan of care is for the day. In fact, everyone helped create the assessment and plan. As people leave, there is a sense of closeness among people that is evident in looks, gestures, and the way people linger for a moment or say goodbye as they go.

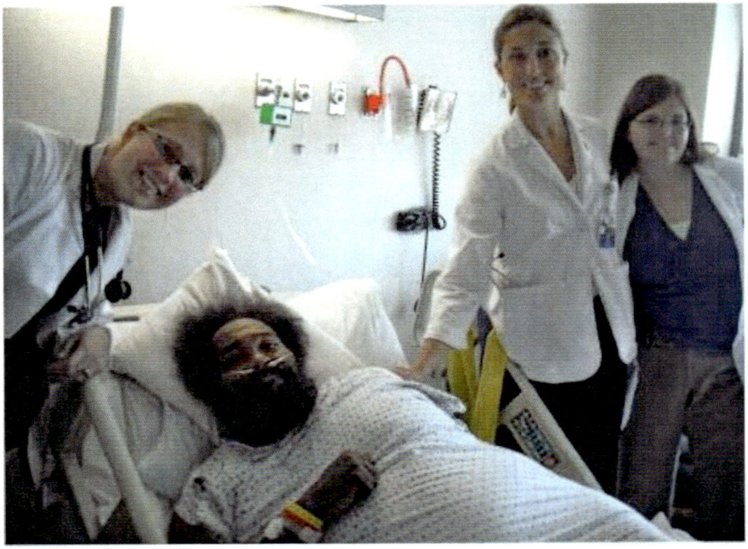

Figure: Collaborative Care – patient and students

A Turning Point

In our experience, there is a turning point for many care teams regarding collaborative care and patient and family participation in rounds and other care activities.

Prior to this turning point, the professional members of the care team are likely to view the purpose of their interactions with patients and family members as being primarily about respectfully gathering information, such as taking a careful history, making and implementing therapeutic decisions, informing the patient and family about the patient's situation and what is being done, and educating the patient and family about the patient's condition.

On the other side of this turning point, there is a different kind of relationship with patients and family members. Perhaps the easiest way to describe this shift is by saying that the patient and family members are included as people, and are "part of the care team" rather than separate from it as the focus of its attention.

As a care team begins to function in this different way, the thoughts, goals, hopes, concerns and expertise of patients and families become much stronger parts of the mix – their thoughts, goals, and concerns are woven throughout the conversations, actions, decisions and plans that are being created together.

In a similar way, there is a turning point regarding what teamwork means for the professional care team. Prior to this shift, members of the care team function independently from one another within their professional roles, with points of overlap and connection such as phone calls and orders. After the turning point, the professional team is much more interdependent and mutually engaged, truly interactive in its work together.

It takes time and firsthand experience for most health professionals to recognize these differences and to appreciate what becomes possible because of these shifts. Until recently, the only kind of care that most people have been trained in or experienced is the traditional model. Usual ways of working feel very natural in health care after years of training, and carry emotional underpinnings of professional and personal identities.

It is important to recognize and honor that both before and after these shifts, the intent of the professional members of the care team is to be respectful of one another and to be respectful and inclusive with patients and family members. These are deep values of professional health care in any model.

When health care professionals working in the traditional way say, "We do that already" about collaborative care, they say this because they are speaking from these deep values. In our research we see a commitment to the care of patients on every service we observe. We respect this commitment. What is different about collaborative care is how this commitment is operationalized. Standing in the traditional world, the differences are not easy to see. For patients, though, the changes are striking.

In collaborative care the flow of interactions is much more level and participatory than in traditional care, with a different kind of active engagement by everyone present, including patients and family members. There is an observably different sense of power and information sharing, and a different kind of team learning.

The interactions of collaborative care happen at a team level and are notably more than the sum of individual actions. The nature and meaning of care change in collaborative care. There is a central focus on the patient as a person, a commitment to inviting people into shared work together, and a belief that new ideas will be found when a team works together collaboratively.

What you can see later will be different

These distinctions will become more evident as your team gains experience with collaborative care. You will start to see things with new insights. What you begin to see will surprise you.

We encourage you to come back to these descriptions from time to time, as a way of reflecting about what you may be able to see later, and as a measure of what you have learned. Our own journey was like that. With each advance we were startled to look back at how much we were not seeing before, even though we thought we were. With each step you will be able to see more.

Throughout the *Field Guide to Collaborative Care* we hope to make these distinctions even more evident, and to illuminate the field shifts that are necessary for collaborative care to be successfully established and sustained.

In summary, the observable differences between traditional practice and collaborative care are significant. The box below highlights some of the most notable distinctions. These differences will be discussed in greater detail in following sections.

Traditional health care practice 1) is based in the individual work of practitioners in professional roles; 2) has gradients of authority and is hierarchically organized; 3) is centered on treating or preventing disease as defined from scientific and professional perspectives; 4) relies on notes, orders and other methods of explicit direction and communication to achieve coordination and goal orientation among professional roles and disciplines (patients and families are not usually active participants in this process); and 5) locates power and decision making primarily in health care practitioners according to their professional roles.

Alternatively,

Collaborative care 1) is based in the collective work of interprofessional teams including patients and family members as active participants in care and decision making; 2) is participatory and inquiry-based – inviting, welcoming and utilizing the expertise of patients, families, and practitioners; 3) is centered on what has meaning for people through strengths, values and contributions of each participant, including yet going beyond disease treatment and prevention; 4) utilizes a mixture of explicit communication and rich tacit knowledge in an intentionally-developed context of ongoing shared experiences, reflective conversations, and team-level learning to achieve coordination and goal orientation among all participants, including patients and families; and 5) distributes power and decision making among all involved by acknowledging and deferring to expertise and leadership from multiple sources.

PART TWO

IMPLEMENTATION ROAD MAP

- Every Care Environment is Unique

- Preparing
  Activating
  Deepening
  Sustaining

- Activity Flows and Timeline

- Using the Collaborative Care Toolkit

- Assessing Progress – Five Frames View

Every Care Environment is Unique

Have you ever noticed that different care areas, places that are a lot alike in many other ways, often have different personalities? Over here, on this floor, people are always smiling. They are busy, but there is no sense of burden in their busyness. Over here, though, on this other floor, there is a different feeling in the air. It's not bad; actually, both floors are good places. But something is different somehow about this place compared to that one. Sometimes the differences wear you down, and sometimes they lift you up. You can sense it when you step off the elevator.

This book is about the benefits of these differences. It is about how to intentionally build collaborative care environments filled with collective knowledge and a sense of "aliveness" of the human spirit – differences that make giving and receiving care in these special places remarkably rewarding, safe, and effective.

In order to make these differences between environments easier to see and talk about, we have developed a term for what you feel when you step off the elevator. We call it a "social field."

Our definition of a social field is:

A living collective intelligence of accumulated experiences, memories, and connections that grows over time among members of a team who are able to work together regularly and reflect together about their interactions.

That is a lot, so take a minute and read it again, slowly...

A social field is...a living collective intelligence...of accumulated experiences, memories, and connections...that grows over time... among members of a team...who are able to work together regularly...and reflect together about their interactions.

Picture a social field as a living memory bubble hovering over a care environment. The memory bubble contains the accumulated experiences, stories, and connections of the people who have created them there over time. That living social field is what you feel when you walk into that care environment.

From our experience and research, we think that the idea of social fields is really useful. We believe the abilities of exceptional teams are developed and applied in social fields.

If you want to read more about social fields, skip to the last part of this book where we talk much more about them. But for now, it is enough to envision and remember this central idea about social fields: *what happens among people creates a lingering effect that has an impact on what happens next.*

Consider two care teams.

One team is trying to start collaborative care as a best practice that leaders want to implement. A directive is passed down: beginning on a certain day, team training begins. After that, the team will be accountable for making daily bedside rounds, with all professions together and patients and families present.

A second team also wants to implement collaborative care, but goes about it in a different way. People are invited to weekly meetings where they are able to talk and reflect with other people they work with. Each person is given an opportunity to talk about what is important to them. The team is given time to consider how they might care for patients even more effectively by working together in new ways. Interprofessional care with active engagement of patients and families is discussed as a goal. The team continues to meet and talk regularly, then progresses to simulations, and finally to collaborative care. Weekly meetings continue as the team studies and refines their new care routines.

In our experience, the first team is likely to have a difficult and disappointing experience. The "best practice" of collaborative daily bedside rounds probably won't work as intended and may not last very long, if it even begins at all. The second team has a much greater likelihood of success.

Look closely at the success of the second team. How is their success being created? The capabilities needed for collaborative care are being constructed in their meetings and conversations, as people figure out together what to do, and how to do it. Also, the meetings and conversations are a place where people can test and try out new ideas and approaches, allowing the new ways to begin to make new sense and have greater meaning for people.

The difference between these two approaches is more than giving people time to "buy in" to collaborative care. In our experience, buying in isn't how it works. Buying in implies that someone is selling something. People need to be invited into collaborative care. They need time and opportunities and reasons to create collaborative care together. Our research suggests that the remarkable goodness of collaborative care is "co-created" over time as a team works and learns together, trying out new ideas, modifying how they work together, and building new capabilities.

Think about the last time you were engaged in importing a tool or a practice into the work of your team. What did you do? How did it go?

The success of any change depends on the resources available in the social field in which the change is introduced. Some teams are more willing and able to adopt new practices than others, because in some way before, they have acquired certain abilities. If your team doesn't have the ability to learn and change in your social field, implementing collaborative care will be a different experience than if you have built that ability already.

Social fields carry a sense of "oughtness," which is an expression of how people in the social field make sense of things, and what has meaning for them. If a proposed new practice makes sense and has meaning for people in your care environment, the new practice is likely to be adopted. Conversely, if something new doesn't make sense or doesn't have meaning for people, it is likely to be overtly or covertly ignored at first. For example, if an appreciation for engaging patients and family in care is already alive and thriving in your care environment, a proposal to implement collaborative care will be met with a very different response than if this is an unfamiliar idea.

Further, even if a proposed practice makes sense, people may not feel they have the power to make the change. Part of the oughtness of a social field concerns perceptions of power and patterns of decision making. For example, it may make sense to many people to talk in ordinary language on rounds with patients and families, but who in a particular care environment feels they have the power to change that? Implementation strategies for collaborative care need to account for these realities. Although providing evidence and education about a proposed new practice can help shape what is possible, it is the "response" in the social field to the proposed changes that determines what happens next.

Remember that your care environment is unique, and that the responses you will see are meaning-based, and deeply rooted in prior experience and the specific local history of your care team.

In our experience, collaborative care is successfully implemented team-by-team, one local environment at a time, as new collective capabilities are built and developed. The special capabilities of collaborative care, including the capabilities that underlie reliability and resilience, are locally produced and have significance in special ways in each particular care environment.

As our colleague Jeff Brown said one day with a wry smile, "So what our research is showing is that 'the wheel truly needs to be reinvented every time'." We increasingly know that he is right.

Sometimes, with a goal of efficiency, it is tempting to look for pathways for change that do not require reinventing the wheel. Leaders may look for best practices to import, with an expectation that the new practices themselves, put in place, will produce the same benefits here that they did in the environment where they were first developed. There is a tendency to focus on the practices themselves, rather than on the work of implementing the practices, as what makes the difference – the source of the magic.

We have learned to view this differently. We encourage care teams to focus on the implementation activities underlying collaborative care as the true best practice, as much or more than the collaborative care processes themselves. Collaborative care is implemented and sustained through meetings, conversations, reflections, and collective learning over time. The actions for implementing collaborative care involve resetting and restructuring the care environment so these happen in new ways.

The work that brings collaborative care to life is what produces its benefits. In each unique local environment, implementing collaborative care requires time, patience and thoughtful structural changes, and is ongoing. To quote a familiar expression, collaborative care is "not a one walk dog."

Implementing collaborative care involves intentionally reshaping the care environment in ways that create new kinds of generative interactions, which in turn allows the new patterns of collaborative care to emerge, and meanings to shift.

Once these changes have begun, a development process is set in motion. Ongoing cycles of action and reflection generate increasing resources for collaborative care in your social field.

Implementation happens differently in every care environment, with specifics that are not entirely predictable, yet can be intentionally nurtured. To achieve success, your strategies, plans, sequencing, pacing, measurements, and expectations need to account for this organic, non-linear, emergent nature of uptake and development.

Preparing – Activating – Deepening – Sustaining

The *Field Guide to Collaborative Care* is arranged in parts. The parts immediately following this overview section are called Preparing, Activating, Deepening, and Sustaining. Each part refers to an implementation step along the developmental pathway of a collaborative care environment. The steps are designed to establish and develop a care environment that is filled with awareness, trust, and learning. Each step is described in greater detail later in the Field Guide, but here is the overview:

Preparing is an important initial step that sets the stage for the emergence of collaborative care. This involves establishing preconditions in the care environment that allow a consistent team to work and learn together collaboratively. The preconditions implemented in this step include establishing collaborative leadership that models welcoming, invitation, and engagement; and organizing for teamwork by reconfiguring locations, staffing, and scheduling so people are able to work together consistently.

Activating is a step that brings collaborative care to life in a particular care environment. This involves establishing weekly system meetings; developing these meetings to become the central home for the collaborative care environment; planning and beginning daily collaborative care; and actively engaging patients and families as integral members of the care team. The actions in this step establish collaborative patterns and routines in the care environment that will last long beyond this early stage.

Deepening is ongoing work that continues throughout the life of the collaborative environment. This involves establishing action-reflection learning systems that connect the actions of daily care to opportunities for collective reflection and improvement in weekly systems meetings. This step adds processes and routines for monitoring and improving systems of care as a normal part of work at a front line level, and connects these with processes at the organization level, to improve systems of care at root levels. Reliability and resilience emerge and deepen with this step, as development of the care team accelerates, and ongoing learning and improvement activities progressively elevate and simplify care for professional care team members, patients, and families.

Sustaining is ongoing relational work that further connects and strengthens the collaborative care environment, and manages alignment between the routines and leadership of collaborative care and the more traditional organizational practices of most health care organizations. This involves proactively nurturing connections to the organization and its leaders in ways that create and demonstrate value, including outcomes excellence and reputation; active participation in learning networks, presentations, research, and mentoring; and educational events, simulations, and site visits so leaders, professionals, patients, families, and students can experience and understand collaborative care.

Activity Flows and Timeline

The following diagram offers a summary of the flows, sequencing, and pacing of major activities for establishing collaborative care in a local care environment. This diagram brings together the various sections of the *Field Guide to Collaborative Care* in an overview that can be used to help plan and monitor your implementation efforts.

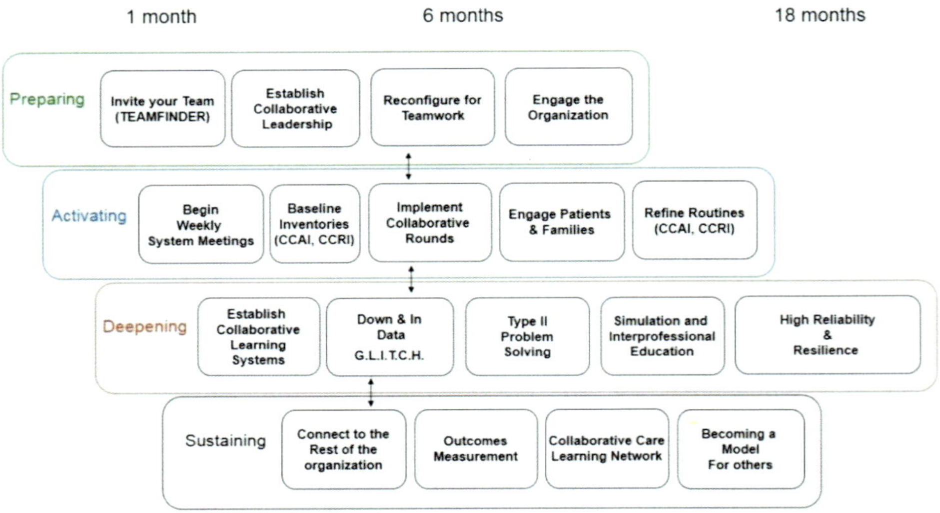

Figure: Activity Flows and Timeline

Do not be surprised if your implementation efforts vary from this general overview. Remember, the "wheel needs to be reinvented every time" in each unique care environment. Your team will have its own uniqueness. Expect that this will happen, and trust your instincts. However, in a general sense we usually see and anticipate the work of implementing collaborative care as taking place over eighteen months in four parallel and connected steps of Preparing, Activating, Deepening and Sustaining.

Each of these steps is described in its own part of the Field Guide. Note that the Activity Flows and Timeline figure mentions using inventories ("TEAMFINDER," "CCAI," "CCRI") as you consider and plan for these activities. These inventories are included in the *Collaborative Care Toolkit* described below.

Using the Collaborative Care Toolkit

The *Collaborative Care Toolkit* is available on-line at www.cca-home.org and in printed form as a companion publication to the *Field Guide to Collaborative Care.* The *Collaborative Care Toolkit* consists of three inventories designed for use by care teams while implementing collaborative care. The inventories in the Toolkit are: the *Collaborative Care TEAMFINDER*, *Collaborative Care Activation Inventory (CCAI), and Collaborative Care Resource Inventory (CCRI).*

The Toolkit offers your care team a structured way to take stock of your current collaborative care environment and decide what to do next. The inventories included in the Toolkit can be used as guides to self-assess and check in on progress over time. They can also be used as qualitative and quantitative instruments that can help your team assess progress from baseline measures.

We encourage you to use the *Collaborative Care Toolkit* as a guide, reference and conversation starter early on as you begin to implement collaborative care, and to keep coming back to the Toolkit as you go along. Implementing collaborative care is a process of ongoing discovery that will make increasing sense as you gain more and more experience working in these ways. The Toolkit will allow your team to see the progress you are making.

We will briefly describe each inventory in the Toolkit.

The Collaborative Care TEAMFINDER

The Collaborative Care TEAMFINDER invites your team to consider the kinds of patients you care for, the settings in which care is given, and for each setting, the ideal roles and connections of your team at its best. The TEAMFINDER is useful as people begin to look beyond their individual professional roles and start to envision the entire interprofessional team.

In our experience, most people in health care don't usually view their work from the perspective of an entire interprofessional team. For example, when invited to talk about teamwork, nurses often talk about their unit and the other nurses they work with; physicians often describe their practices and partners, or the fellows, residents, and medical students they work with; and so on. People talk this way because traditional work environments are organized this way. Collaborative care requires a larger view.

The TEAMFINDER is designed to help people think across their usual boundaries, visualizing the entire interprofessional team, including other health professions, and patients and families. It is also useful for helping people begin to look beyond their immediate care settings, such as a floor, OR, or ICU, to a larger picture of care for patients with a particular pattern of need, and to consider what optimum connections would look like between various parts of the care environment.

The Collaborative Care TEAMFINDER is especially useful as your care team begins inviting people to participate in your collaborative care initiative. It is also useful as you envision the "natural work cluster" of roles that you hope will begin to work especially well together; and how well your care environment is organized, and might be better organized, to support teamwork.

The Collaborative Care Activation Inventory (CCAI)

The Collaborative Care Activation Inventory (CCAI) invites your team to self-assess a set of preconditions in your care environment that we have identified as important for the emergence of collaborative care. The CCAI helps your team identify and strengthen these preconditions. Each precondition is described in a narrative paragraph. Your team is then asked to consider and rate ten sub-descriptions about each precondition from the perspective of your own care environment. The ratings are totaled and a score for each precondition is then transferred to a diagram that allows your team to visualize which preconditions are well developed in your care environment, and which are not.

The Collaborative Care Activation Inventory (CCAI) is a condensed reference, checklist, and action guide for implementing collaborative care. The CCAI will help your team understand and navigate the action steps for implementing the Social Field Model of Collaborative Care. We recommend using the CCAI relatively early on in your work, and coming back to it often as a way of assessing your progress and asking what to do next.

We believe that implementing collaborative care is like growing a garden; the CCAI is designed to be useful for assessing and optimizing the growing conditions. If the preconditions for collaborative care are strongly in place in a care environment, collaborative care is highly likely to emerge and develop there.

If there are preconditions that are not well developed in your care environment, and your team would like to strengthen them, the CCAI is useful as a guide for action as well as for assessment. By returning to the sub-descriptions for a particular precondition, each sub-description can be read as a specific action step that can be taken to strengthen that precondition.

The Collaborative Care Resource Inventory (CCRI)

The Collaborative Care Resource Inventory (CCRI) invites your team to consider and self-assess eight contextual resources – capabilities available in your social field – that we have identified as highly characteristic of evolved collaborative care environments. Each resource is described by a narrative paragraph that has been developed from interviews with actual collaborative care teams. Using these, your team is invited to reflect about these resources in your own care environment.

Another way of thinking about the resources described in the CCRI is: "things that really great collaborative care teams can do, that less developed teams aren't able to do yet." Collaborative care grows and becomes more capable as these contextual resources are built and developed in your care environment.

Our experience with teams using the CCRI is that people often view the resources described in the CCRI as goals they agree they would like to achieve, but that seem out of reach when they first take the inventory. Later, however, as they come back to the inventory, teams are usually surprised and pleased how much progress has been made. Resources that seemed out of reach at first can now be envisioned, or may already be in place.

We recommend using the CCRI relatively early on, as a way for your team to imagine and begin thinking about these resources. As your collaborative care initiative progresses, you may want to come back to the CCRI at regular intervals, so your team can be reminded of these resources as goals, and as a way of assessing progress toward achieving them. The CCRI can be useful just as a conversation starter, and it can also be used as a quantitative assessment instrument. Suggestions for using the CCRI as a group activity are included as part of the inventory.

Putting it all together –The Social Field Model

The CCAI helps your team assess *preconditions* that we believe are important for the emergence and development of collaborative care, in the figure below on the left; and the CCRI helps your team assess *contextual resources* in your social field that we believe are especially important for achieving reliability and resilience, in the figure below on the right. Collaborative care has a trajectory of growth and development from *Preconditions*, to *Contextual Resources*, to *Reliability and Resilience*. We call this the Social Field Model of Collaborative Care. The last section of the book describes this model in detail, but here is a summary:

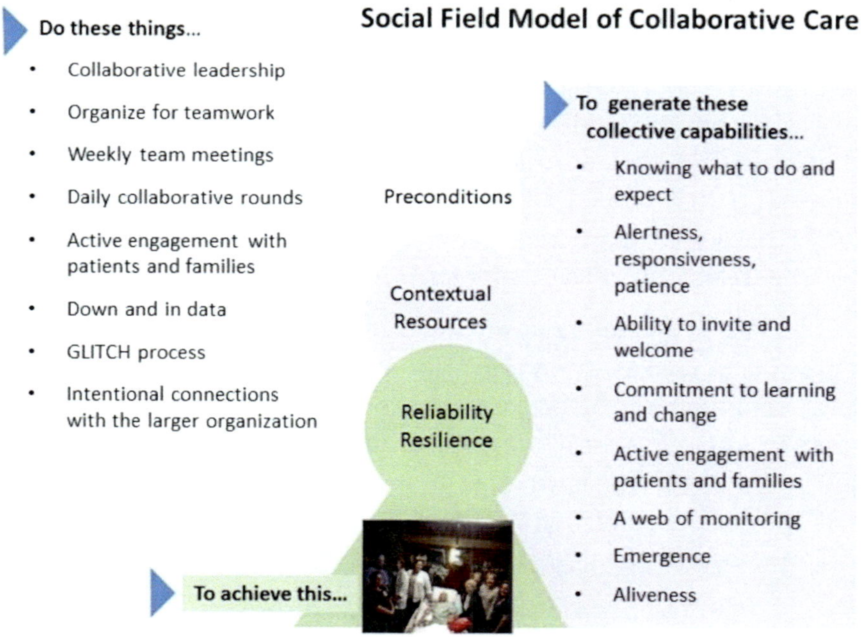

Figure: Preconditions and Contextual Resources of the Social Field Model
"Do these things...to generate these collective capabilities...to achieve this."

Assessing Progress – Five Frames View

It is possible to talk about the steps toward collaborative care as a process of evolution and development that happens in phases over time. Frames are snapshots of the evolving phases. One way of assessing the development of a collaborative care environment is to reflect about the experiences of each Frame.

The reflections organized by Frames are from our research. As with most deep change, the experiences are less linear than depicted and also harder to visualize when you are in it. However, recognizing that you are in a certain Frame may help people understand experiences and manage expectations.

The Frames discussed below are intended to help your team reflect on progress toward collaborative care. The Frames help you understand how your care context is evolving, may evolve in the future, and what you may expect at various times. The Frames may help you see where you are, explain what is happening, and predict what will happen next. For example, using the Frames your team might say, "This is a great Frame 2 story," or, "These stresses are normal for Frame 3. They will get better."

The Frames are also useful for understanding how your organization is likely to respond to the work you are doing in your care environment. Most organizations support work from the perspective of Frame 1, traditional care. Moving toward a stable new norm of collaborative care is likely to require changes in how your organization functions. Visualizing the Frames can help you navigate evolving realities and expectations of your organization.

The Frames are similar to those of any process of deep change. The Five Frames move from an existing status quo, through initial interest and curiosity, to the hard work of making changes, to local acceptance and belief, and finally to a new way of working that is fully integrated and supported organizationally.

The figure below illustrates the five Frames of the journey to collaborative care.

Frame 1	Frame 2	Frame 3	Frame 4	Frame 5
Professional Providers	The Invitation	The Shift	A Guarded Fragile New life	A New Place of Caring
Acting from professional roles (traditional care) Patients' ask: "Don't you people talk to each other?"	Acting from a sense of awakening curiosity "How can we do even better?"	Acting from a spirit of trying to learn and change " We have to keep a foot in both worlds for now."	Acting from a new appreciation for collaborative care "Collaborative care is our expectation AND is still at risk."	Acting from a new context for care "This is the only way we know."

Figure: Five Frames of the journey to collaborative care

Frame 1 – Professional Providers

Frame 1 is traditional care. Each profession has its own understanding of the needs of the patient, and works from that understanding. There is some connection of professional workflows related to patient care in Frame 1, but workflows are not coordinated as interdependent. Providers work from the perspectives of their professional roles and connect with others as needed. Patients and families are viewed as recipients or consumers of professional expertise. Health care professionals know what to do in this Frame. This is how most health professionals have been trained and practice. People try hard to provide good care despite increasingly difficult expectations and stresses. Patients ask, "Don't you people talk to each other?"

Frame 2 – The Invitation

In Frame 2 an invitation is made for something better. Most practitioners don't realize that their work could be done differently, but a few people begin to say, "Oh my gosh! We can do better than this." In Frame 2 a few people begin to talk, try new approaches, and start to see the possibility of something new. A seed is planted. Hope begins. A collaborative care initiative begins. There is excitement and also a sense of risk. The feeling is, "OK, I'm willing to try this, but it doesn't fit with the rest of my work life." There is hesitancy about the new ways except among a few early advocates. These advocates are comfortable taking risks and often don't see the risks, just the potential. Patients and families who are able to participate recognize the benefits immediately. Their new happiness makes people take notice.

Frame 3 – The Shift (hard work)

A growing number of people begin to participate in the new collaborative routines, which are still considered experimental. Most people aren't willing to let go of the old entirely, but some are willing to put in the extra energy needed to try the new. Most people try the new and also hold on to the old patterns, moving back and forth as the need arises. The thought is, "OK, maybe this isn't going away. But I need to keep a foot in both worlds." For newcomers the changes are easier, because the new patterns make intuitive sense. Aliveness of the human spirit is showing up now, and people can sense and feel the excitement. The old context is less influential, which is threatening for some. There is growing excitement among a group of believers, cautious interest by many, and criticism, even ridicule, by naysayers. This is a time of hard work and cautious hope. It is a puzzling time – familiar routines are no longer certain; new routines are not fully in place.

Frame 4 – A Guarded, Fragile New Life (still at risk)

This is experienced as a peak time. People in the care environment increasingly understand and trust the new routines and the new rules of what it means to work this way. The pull of the old is still there at times, but the center of work now is clearly the new collaborative care routines with active engagement of patients and families. People function as a true team now and are able to fill in for each other. Guidance no longer comes from individual professional care plans. Other departments are aware. Collaborative care is ON the radar. It is normal now to work this way here, but not elsewhere. The unit teaches newcomers these ways, saying, "This is how we do things around here." The experiences of people working in Frame 4 makes progression to Frame 2 and Frame 3 possible for others. People are becoming comfortable again and life is simpler. Collaborative care has become an expectation, yet it remains organizationally fragile. The changes do not have full support and commitment yet outside of the care environment. The environment still requires protection by a strong leader, or by research or pilot status. People here know the benefits, but others may be threatened. The organization must respond, either by changing itself, or by stopping the initiative.

Frame 5 – A New Place of Caring

The organization is designed and operated to support this. The care environment is structured this way. People are employed this way, and are trained this way. They say, "This is the only way we do our work." "This is what we expect as practitioners, and it is what patients and families expect." "It is our only routine." "This way of working is the only thing we do." Leaders support it. No sanctioning or protection is required. The incongruence is gone. (Authors' note: We haven't seen Frame 5 yet.)

PART THREE

PREPARING

- Preconditions and Emergence
- Foundational Preconditions
    - Collaborative Leadership
    - Organizing for Teamwork
- Keeping the Focus on:
  "What will make this possible?"

Preconditions and Emergence

One of the biggest surprises in our own journey toward collaborative care was the realization that collaborative care is an emergent phenomenon. We have found that it is surprisingly hard to create a collaborative care environment by focusing on collaborative care directly, yet remarkably effective to do so by shifting attention and implementation efforts to the preconditions from which collaborative care emerges.

Early in our experience we based our efforts to implement collaborative care on descriptions of exceptional teamwork. It made sense that if we learned about these principles and techniques and then implemented them, our care would improve.

We developed a relationship with an expert in aviation safety and high reliability teamwork and worked diligently to implement this theoretical knowledge. We wrote about this when we received the Eisenberg Award. We were convinced that the improved outcomes our team was experiencing were due to these principles and techniques, primarily in collaborative rounds.

It didn't work out quite that way. As others read our work and tried to implement collaborative rounds as their first action, their experiences and outcomes usually did not match ours. It never occurred to us that the improvements we were experiencing could be due to other things that we were not considering.

During some of our early work we had worked closely with another care team that was interested in replicating our approach to care. Many members of that care team had spent time working side-by-side with us as they were preparing to establish a new program. Several years later we reconnected with them.

The leaders of the new program were excited to have us visit. They looked forward to showing us their program and their outcomes, which equaled or exceeded our own. We were excited, too. The difficulties other teams were having replicating our work based on our writings weighed heavily in our thoughts as we prepared to visit this remarkably successful program. We wondered, what were they doing that made their efforts successful, when so many others were having problems?

Much of what we had written focused on the routines of collaborative rounds. Shortly after we arrived for our research visit one of us said to the physician leader of the successful program, "We can't wait to see your collaborative rounds." The leader seemed genuinely surprised. He turned to us with a puzzled look and said, "Rounds?" He paused and then said, "Oh, you must think that collaborative rounds is the reason our outcomes are so good. I guess the rounds do matter, but for us what makes all the difference is the weekly team meetings."

"Weekly team meetings?" we asked. "Yes," he said, "just like you showed us, we have weekly system meetings of our entire care team every week. In the meetings we are able to sit down together, talk about how we're doing, get to know each other really well, and figure out together how we can do an even better job. It is the center of our work together."

We were astonished. We had not recognized until that moment how important the weekly team meetings were. We hadn't understood that our reflections together as a team in the weekly meetings were so important for the success of the daily bedside rounds and many other elements of our program.

After this visit our approach shifted. Gradually we began to understand that collaborative care is much more than making rounds together. We began to view collaborative care as a deeper "field shift" in how people relate, work, and learn together.

The more we studied collaborative care, the more we began to see that collaborative care depends on the development of meaningful connections among people, and on the growth of new team-level capabilities enabled by those connections.

Moreover, we began to recognize that the connections and capabilities underlying collaborative care can be intentionally nurtured, and that the development of these connections and capabilities can be activated and supported by assuring that conditions are right for this to happen.

We began to identify a set of "preconditions" in the care environment that, when intentionally introduced and thoughtfully strengthened, make the emergence and development of collaborative care highly likely. This was a major reorientation for us and is now central to our understanding of collaborative care.

Grow it like a garden

The Social Field Model views collaborative care as something that is highly likely to grow and develop naturally in a care environment if conditions are right for that.

A garden metaphor is useful. A thoughtful gardener focuses on establishing optimum growing conditions: working the soil, providing the right nutrients, assuring proper moisture and sunlight. When these are attended to carefully, the garden is highly likely to flourish.

We believe implementing collaborative care is just like that. The Social Field Model encourages a care team to consider the nature of its care environment and to intentionally strengthen preconditions that are conducive to the emergence and development of collaborative care. The implementation focus is the care environment. Collaborative care is implemented by optimizing the care environment in ways that strengthen and support collaborative interactions of the care team as a whole.

This is done by assuring there is collaborative leadership that builds trust and encourages curiosity, excellence, integrity, and engagement; by organizing the care environment with teamwork in mind so the entire care team can work consistently together; by establishing routines as a normal part of their work together that make it possible for the care team to reflect, learn, and continuously monitor and improve the systems they rely on; and by carefully connecting the local care environment to the larger organization to optimize effectiveness and sustainability.

This approach, of viewing collaborative care as something that emerges when conditions are right, and of implementing collaborative care by intentionally strengthening preconditions, is a central point of understanding of the Social Field Model.

In this section, Preparing, we discuss two preconditions that from our practice and research we believe are foundational for the emergence and development of collaborative care. We call these foundational because everything else rests upon them. After discussing these two foundational preconditions, in other parts we describe six additional preconditions we believe are helpful for Activating, Deepening, and Sustaining collaborative care.

The foundational preconditions for collaborative care are 1) *collaborative leadership*, which is an approach to leadership that distributes power and expertise throughout the care environment, and 2) *organizing for teamwork*, which means intentionally co-locating, organizing, staffing and scheduling the care environment to support the emergence and development of collaborative care.

Foundational Precondition – Collaborative Leadership

The first foundational precondition is collaborative leadership. A special kind of leadership is required to implement and develop a collaborative care environment. Remember that the new ways of working together that develop as your care team implements collaborative care will last long after the original team members have gone. What the initial leadership is like will be reflected in everything else that happens in the care environment.

In our experience, successful collaborative leaders are respected and admired for their clinical abilities, and for a steadfast commitment to excellence which shows consistently in their work. They have a natural inclination to be respectful and inclusive, and to treat people with dignity. They have a low need for personal control, and a high interest in seeking out, honoring, and developing the expertise and leadership abilities of others.

Collaborative leaders look beyond the immediate moment of care, to the care environment itself. They recognize that every action they take has an effect on others around them that shapes the care environment – either strengthening it or taking away the capacity of the care environment to grow and develop. Collaborative leaders choose their actions carefully to intentionally build and develop the esteem and expertise of others around them, and to enhance the capability of the care environment. One collaborative leader said, "My goal is to make myself unneeded."

It is important to recognize that the attitudes and skills of collaborative leadership can be learned and intentionally adopted. Some of the best collaborative leaders did not start out that way. They began as individual leaders, intensely committed to caring for their patients, and developed new abilities for collaborative leadership later, when they recognized how valuable these are.

From "Who leads?" to "What is accomplished?"

There are interesting conversations in the literature about the question, "Who should lead the collaborative team?"

In our experience, the most effective pattern of initial leadership for collaborative care is joint leadership by admired RN/MD leaders who clearly respect and enjoy each other, and who work well with others across all professions. Collaborative leaders encourage and model leadership that is fluid and moves from person to person and role to role based on strengths and expertise rather than positional authority. It is noteworthy how often early modeling of collaborative leadership may come from any person across the team. We have seen exceptional early adoption and modeling of collaborative leadership by social workers, pharmacists, chaplains, physical therapists and physical therapy assistants, nurse practitioners, administrators, physician assistants, patients, family members, and many others.

The important point is that collaborative leadership starts with individuals, but quickly becomes more than an individual attribute. Collaborative leadership builds the capacities of an entire care team to jointly create a care environment that is respectful, inclusive, confident and generative.

In collaborative leadership, the team itself becomes capable and powerful, rather than any one person or role. This shift from individual leaders to leadership as a collective capability can be puzzling at first. But once it becomes clear that the team itself is the central actor, all sorts of possibilities become available.

From a collaborative leadership perspective, every role is important and leads at various times. What matters is not who leads, but rather, what collaborative leadership accomplishes.

Leading toward a state of generativity

Collaborative leadership is generative. Very often what is created through collaboration cannot be known with certainty beforehand by the people whose collaboration makes the new things possible. Collaborative leadership reaches out toward the new, and takes pleasure in growth, change, and ongoing renewal.

Collaborative leaders feel and project wholeness in situations that by their nature are necessarily full of ambiguity and uncertainties. Collaboration does not mean consensus. It means being able to account for differences while going forward together.

Collaborative leadership is authentically curious about multiple viewpoints in appreciative ways. Collaborative leadership "holds space" that allows differences to be safely and respectfully recognized and valued, and for something new to emerge.

Leading into the unknown

Collaborative leaders move forward into the unknown together with vision and belief, creating and maintaining a safe place where people can do the difficult, rewarding work of trying something new, improving it, and eventually making it their own.

Collaborative leaders are willing to say, "Let's try this. Together we can figure this out."

The primary tools of collaborative leadership are careful listening, patience, adaptability, persistence, and courage that others can take comfort in when nothing seems secure or certain.

Leading toward a more level hierarchy

Collaborative leadership requires and causes a leveling of hierarchy. Collaborative leaders are comfortable standing beside others, and often in the service of others, rather than standing before them. This requires finding satisfaction in guiding, nurturing, and supporting more than in directing.

Growth of leadership capacity and role modeling

It is important to recognize the symbolic nature of collaborative leadership and the far-reaching effects of role modeling. Collaborative leadership is learned by watching others. The symbolic effects of kindness, patience, listening, and authentic respect are profound. These do not have to be explicitly taught. They are leaned best from experience, by example.

As people watch and learn from collaborative leaders, it is not so much the events themselves, but the response to the events from which the greatest lessons are learned. Thoughtfulness, integrity, humility, and constancy of purpose are the responses that create the deepest and longest lasting effects.

Collaborative leaders find their greatest satisfaction in watching their leadership become less and less necessary as their work comes alive in the shared accomplishments of many others.

Careful attention to the human spirit

Most importantly, collaborative leadership carefully accounts for and honors the human spirit at its best.

The starting point of collaborative leadership is an unshakable belief in the desire of every person in health care to do their best. This can be counted on. It is the fundamental assumption in collaborative care. Everything is built from that, and every course correction orients around that. The human spirit, and the dedication to patient care that flows from it, is the North Star.

Collaborative care is an extension of the human spirit, and must be invited into being with respect and patience.

Defining moments

The history of a collaborative care initiative will have a handful of defining moments with regard to leadership. The most important of these will be times when a few people have an awareness of something with crystal clarity, yet others either cannot see or are unwilling to see what these few can. These moments – which are rare but always seem to occur – will either shatter the emerging collaboration or take it to new levels.

There is no greater test of collaborative leadership than these moments. Collaborative leaders will know in these moments with every fiber of their being that something needs to be done in a particular way – and yet others at that moment are either unable or unwilling to move in that direction.

Such moments are authentic tests of collaborative leaders. By remaining true to a vision, yet doing so with humility expressed in actions, collaborative leaders establish even deeper bonds of connection and respect with and among the collaborative team.

The only effective response for collaborative leaders in such moments is to clearly state the desired direction, and at the same time to remain united with the others, yielding into the path that others are able or willing to take.

The decisive act of yielding at these moments – out of insightful and respectful strength, not weakness – is one of the most fascinating paradoxes of collaborative leadership. From these few yet powerful tests, an environment of trust is created.

Acknowledging the crucible

People engaged in the care of patients are working in a crucible. They are highly focused, stressed, and functioning in deeply held thought and work patterns often inseparable from their personal identities. It is not easy in such an environment to ask people to consider trying new things.

Collaborative leaders recognize and respect this crucible and the tensions inherent in trying new ways of providing care. The stress of trying new ways can be managed carefully and thoughtfully so that people remain receptive and continue to function well. Steps forward must be measured enough for that.

The costs and rewards of collaborative leadership

Collaborative leadership does not produce easy rewards. In fact, the costs of collaborative leadership can be very high.

The storms and emotions of human politics have two distinct time cycles, short term and long term. The short term cycles have significant peaks and valleys. Someone may be in today and out tomorrow, a hero one moment and left standing alone and broken the next, as the short term cycles ebb and flow.

The rewards of collaborative leadership are rarely found in short term cycles except among a few very close friends and colleagues willing to stand side by side despite the inherent risks and inevitable losses of leading transformational change. For many others, in fact most, the risks and costs are just too great.

Don't be discouraged by the short term cycles. It is the longer term cycles that matter and endure. The longer term cycles are built from persistence, consistency, and integrity, through incremental actions over years and decades, sometimes more.

Collaborative leadership finds its validation and true measure in the longer term cycles. The rewards and satisfactions of collaborative leadership come over time, often with a depth of human connection and meaning never forgotten over lifetimes.

Summary of things your team can do to increase collaborative leadership

The characteristics of collaborative leadership can be intentionally learned and adopted by anyone in the care environment. Collaborative leadership grows as a collective attribute from the attitudes and actions of people that others watch, learn with, respect and admire. People who lead collaboratively may be formal leaders, informal leaders, and others at all levels.

- You can put in place joint RN/MD/Administrative leadership of your unit by leaders who clearly respect and enjoy each other, and who work well with others across all professions.

- You can strive to establish a leadership environment where everyone together, including patients and families, makes joint decisions about your unit, rather than being directed by an individual person.

- You can encourage and model leadership that is fluid and moves from person to person at particular moments – based on strengths and expertise rather than positional authority.

- Your team can help establish a pattern of leadership "from all levels," with formal leaders present and engaged, but others often contributing expertise, facilitating and presiding.

- Your team can devote effort to welcoming, inviting, and encouraging people to participate in working together, and to find comfort with ambiguity and imperfections while learning.

- You can model honesty and transparency even in the event of mistakes and adverse events, and an emphasis on learning and system improvement over "holding accountable."

- You can intentionally put leadership emphasis on holding space for collective work – expecting the work to be done by all of your team together while maintaining high standards.

- You can emphasize curiosity as an important leadership attribute – encouraging people to ask if we are missing anything, and how we could do an even better job.

- Formal and informal leaders can mentor others toward excellence, in a spirit of helping to guide each other toward a deeper understanding of your collaboration care processes.

- You can intentionally maintain an orientation toward ethics and excellence, with recognition of the importance of each person's work and of small things over time for the long term.

Foundational Precondition – Organizing for Teamwork

The second foundational precondition is organizing for teamwork. In our work we are struck by how often the outcome of an initiative to improve care can be predicted by the structural nature of the care environment. Certain structures are conducive to exceptional care, whereas others are not. In this section we will discuss the organizational structures that we believe are optimal for supporting the emergence of collaborative care.

Patterns of need

In the Social Field Model, the starting point for how to envision care and organize the care environment is something we call "Patterns of Need." A pattern of need is a recurring kind of need for care arising from the nature of the human experience.

For example, a pattern of need that is deeply part of the human experience might be called, "Mothers having babies." Another pattern of need might be called "Outpatient wellness and prevention." A pattern of need that people fortunately do not experience very often anymore might be called, "Polio," and so on.

The spectrum of human experience and the need for care are infinite, but, interestingly, the need for care falls into patterns. These patterns arise from our humanness and the ways we live.

There is a beautiful photograph by nature photographer Fran Halsall that illustrates the co-creative interplay between form and environment. The photograph is of a single tuft of grass growing on a beach. Around the plant a perfect circle has been worn in the sand, traced by the plant as it has blown in the wind.

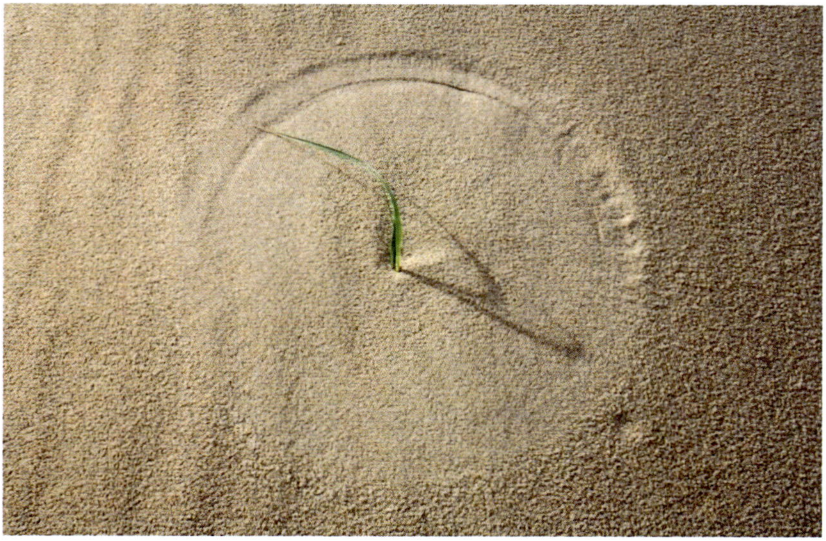

Photo by Fran Halsall: *Mangersta beach, grass circle* (used with permission)
Interactions of form and environment produce patterns

Patterns of need for health care are like the circle in the sand. How we are made as human beings (the tuft of grass), and the ways we live in our environments (the unseen wind), interact to create patterns of need for health care (the circle in the sand).

Patterns of response

Once a pattern of need is identified, the point of interest in health care is how best to respond to it. In contemporary health care, for every pattern of need there is a matching pattern of response – roles and resources that routinely come together to provide the best care possible. The point is not so much the particulars but simply to recognize that care falls in patterns, and with each pattern of need there is a corresponding pattern of response made up of certain predictable roles and resources.

Patterns of need and patterns of response are a helpful way to organize our thinking, and our work, in health care. Of the limitless patterns of need that people experience, a handful – no more – predominate. If the most common patterns of need can be met reliably in exceptional ways, then we are a long way toward creating an even better future for health care.

"Natural work clusters"

Once a pattern of need has been identified and a pattern of response is also recognized, there are many things that can be done to set the stage for care to go really well. We have chosen to call the roles and resources that consistently come together in response to a pattern of need a "natural work cluster."

A "natural work cluster" is basically your ideal care team at its best. It is important to recognize that "natural work clusters" exist, and to be able to see them clearly. This is not always easy to do, because health care is generally not organized around patterns of need or natural work clusters. As will be discussed over the next several pages, a lot of the work of preparing for collaborative care involves intentionally and thoughtfully reorganizing the care environment around patterns of need and natural work clusters to the extent possible.

The concepts of "patterns of need" and "natural work clusters" are closely related to very useful work that has been done about clinical microsystems. The only distinction is that "patterns of need" and "natural work clusters" are idealized conceptual models, useful for visualizing ways of functionally reorganizing and supporting front line care environments.

Visualizing your ideal care team

The Collaborative Care TEAMFINDER is a tool that has been designed to facilitate team discussions about your "natural work cluster." It is intended to help your care team visualize the roles and connections of your team at its best.

The Collaborative Care TEAMFINDER guides your team to think about the patients you care for and the other health care professionals you work with. It then asks you to fill in a template in the TEAMFINDER to visualize your ideal team. We encourage using the TEAMFINDER as a group exercise. As you use the TEAMFINDER, encourage people to think outside of their usual professional framing, and to consider the entire care of the patient.

An example of using the TEAMFINDER template is shown on the next two pages. In order to complete the template, you need to specify the roles and connections of your team at its best. A *role* is an essential part of your team, necessary for doing your best work. A *connection* is a department or service that your team needs to work effectively with to do your best work. Another way of saying this is that roles are right there at the bedside with you, while connections support your work but don't have to be in the room with you to do that.

As you reflect with your care team about the patients you care for and the people you work with, you may realize that your team cares for patients in several settings. For example, a care team that helps mothers have babies may care for patients in birthing rooms, high risk Labor and Delivery, operating room, ICU, triage, and outpatient clinic. Each of these is a setting. The ideal roles and connections of your team may be different in each setting. If your team cares for patients in several settings, work through the Collaborative Care TEAMFINDER for each setting, trying always to keep the bigger picture in mind.

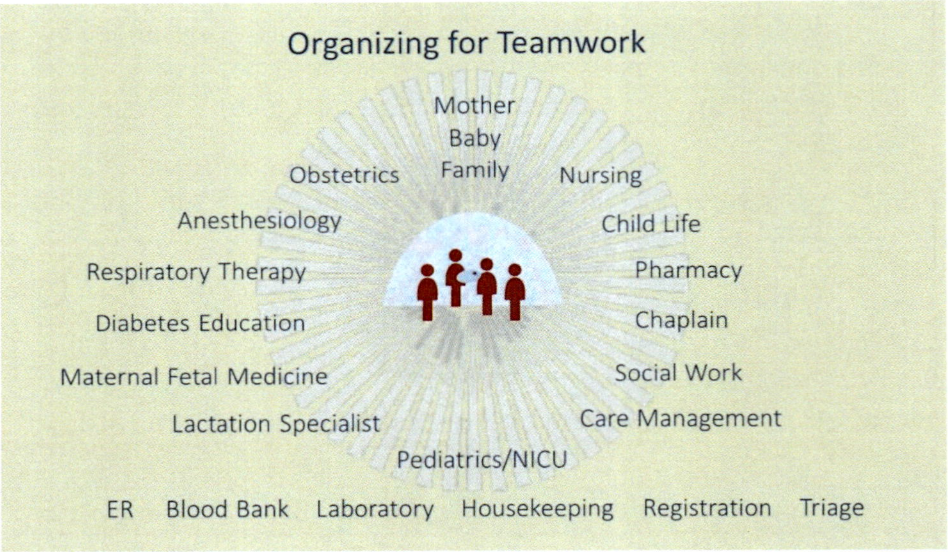

Figure: Example – natural work cluster for mother-baby care

To illustrate how to use the TEAMFINDER, consider the "natural work cluster" of roles and resources in a mother-baby unit at a major metropolitan health center, shown above. Although this picture is nice, it is unlikely that most people working on this unit consider all of these roles together when they think about their work. The TEAMFINDER has been designed to help your care team visualize the roles of your team, then intentionally organize your care environment, staffing, and scheduling so your team can work together at its best in each setting.

The figure below shows a TEAMFINDER template completed for one of the settings of this unit, a birthing room.

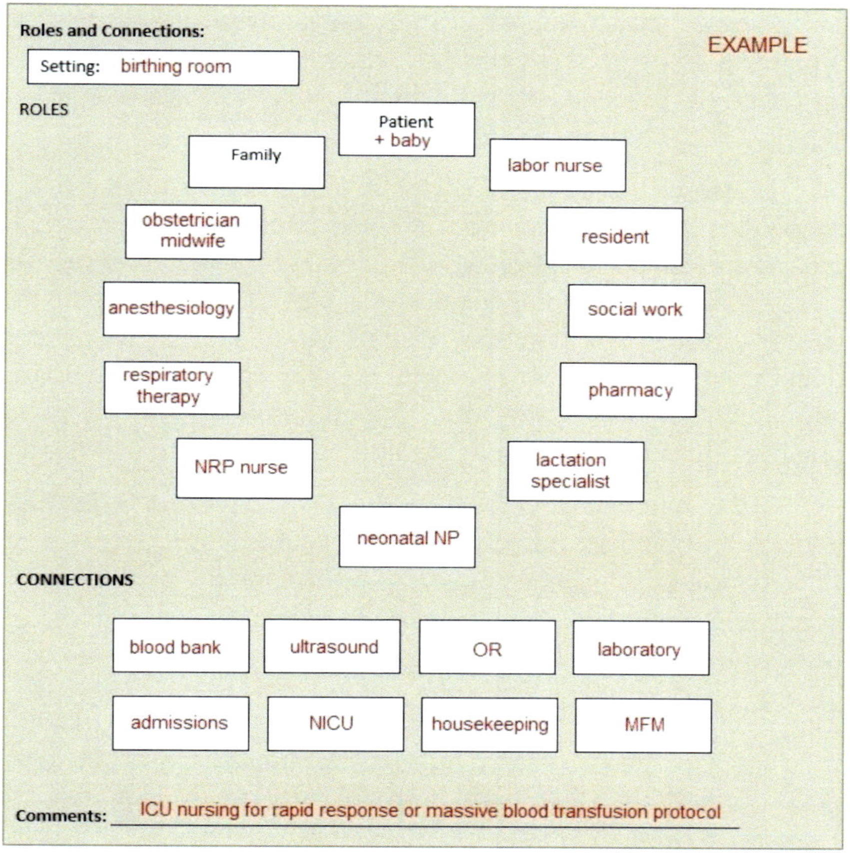

Figure: Example – using the Collaborative Care TEAMFINDER Template
(mother-baby care team in a birthing room setting is illustrated)

The picture of your ideal care team that you develop using the Collaborative Care TEAMFINDER is a helpful starting place for collaborative care. The more you are able to group together the roles of your care team organizationally and functionally, the more success you will have implementing collaborative care.

Organizational boundaries and natural work clusters

How organizational and administrative boundaries are organized in the care environment in support of your ideal team is an important precondition that sets the stage for how easy it is to implement collaborative care.

One of the most significant actions that sets the stage for exceptional collaborative care is being intentional about aligning organizational boundaries with the boundaries of natural work clusters. Organizational boundaries can be established that naturally support a particular pattern of need and a matching pattern of response – for example, co-locating patients needing a certain kind of care, and grouping together with them the people and resources that must work together in response to that need.

We often observe that existing organizational boundaries and work structures do not align well with patterns of need and with natural work clusters. Instead of supporting the patterns of need and response, traditional organizational boundaries and work structures often unintentionally divide and fragment them.

Examples of boundary alignment...or not

Let's consider two familiar examples, one in which organizational boundaries support natural work clusters well, and another where they do not.

For the first example, consider the natural work cluster of roles and resources that comes together in response to a pattern of need of caring for premature infants. In most hospitals this care happens in a specialized neonatal care unit dedicated to those patients. The patients and the people who care for them are co-located in one place. Doctors, nurses, respiratory therapists, pharmacists, social workers, case managers, child life specialists and many other members of the natural work cluster for this pattern of need are likely to work together on a consistent basis.

In contrast, consider a typical internal medicine service in a busy teaching hospital. The natural work cluster of health professionals responding to this pattern of need might include physicians, nurse practitioners, nurses, a case manager, respiratory therapists, social workers, physical therapists, and pharmacists. And of course, the patients and family members.

Yet, in contrast to the natural organizational grouping of people that must work together in the care of premature infants, the natural work cluster of roles and resources caring for internal medicine patients does not often, in our experience, have a co-located organizational home supporting consistent interactions.

Patients may be admitted across many floors wherever a bed is available. Each floor has its own staff of nurses. Respiratory therapists, physical therapists, pharmacists, social workers, case managers and other health professionals may have responsibilities across multiple areas. Their assignments may be made by department, rather than with a view of the natural work cluster in mind. The physician team may be required to move across all of these environments. Without co-location it is much harder to achieve consistency of interaction among team members. The organizational patterns just don't support this.

In the first example of a NICU, it would be relatively easy to implement and strengthen collaborative care because patients are co-located and people are already working consistently together. The way the care environment is organized naturally supports this.

In the second example of med-surg care, it would be difficult to implement and sustain collaborative care without first making structural changes in location, staffing, and scheduling to achieve stability and consistency of interactions. If a performance improvement or collaborative care initiative is introduced, these initiatives are less likely to be successful or long lasting in these environments. The existing organizational structure is not aligned to support them. For many reasons these organizational factors are rarely taken into account in our experience. They are very important, though. They set the stage for making care better.

A couple of stories may be helpful here to illustrate how the care environment can be reorganized with these principles in mind. The first story is about an internal medicine teaching service at a large community hospital – the very circumstance mentioned above. The medical part of the care team on this service consisted of an attending, a senior resident, two first year residents, and two medical students. Patients were admitted to rooms throughout the hospital wherever a bed was available, frequently to five or more different care areas in addition to two ICUs.

Several years earlier it had been recognized that delays in discharges were occurring because of the social complexity of the patients on this service. In response, a social worker and case manager had been assigned to make rounds with the physician team. Also, a pharmacist had been assigned to that care team. Both of these changes were greatly appreciated by everyone involved, and were felt to have been helpful for care.

However, despite these improvements, this particular service had a reputation of being a horrible rotation for the residents and students, and also for nurses, many of whom disliked caring for patients with this team. Nurses felt they were often not being treated respectfully by the medical team, and the medical team was often angry and frustrated because of what were perceived as frequent errors and mistakes made by nurses, who were frequently described as uninterested in providing good care, and borderline incompetent. The everyday working environment on the service was tense and emotionally charged, and nothing seemed to make this any better.

After being introduced to the concept of organizing the care environment for teamwork, the physician leader responsible for this service intentionally began to work more closely with the nursing manager of one of the med-surg floors. Together these leaders were able to successfully change admission policies so that almost all of the non-ICU patients on the service were admitted only to this floor. The physician also relocated the daily report of the medical team to that floor and invited nurses there to participate. Weekly reflective meetings of the entire interprofessional care team were also started.

Very quickly the working environment became noticeably better. Care was perceived to be less stressful, new relationships developed between the nurses and the medical team members, and over time the service developed an entirely better reputation among nurses and medical care team members alike. These changes were felt to be due to new consistencies of interaction that become possible because of the reorganization.

The second story is about a heart surgery program in a small community hospital. Outcomes were poor, and lengths of stay were very long. Patients were kept for extra days in the ICU because of adverse events that were happening after patients left the ICU, while being cared for on a general postoperative floor staffed by nurses who also cared for general surgery, urology, and orthopedic surgery patients. Nurses on this floor would often go many weeks between caring for cardiac surgery patients.

In response to these concerns, changes were made in the organization of the postoperative floor. A four bed dedicated cardiac surgery unit was established on the postoperative floor, demarcated by a natural alcove. This unit, called the Cardio Pulmonary Unit, was staffed by a small cohort of nurses who self-selected to work in the new unit because of their special interest in caring for heart surgery patients. Similarly, a dedicated care team was developed made up of several respiratory therapists, a pharmacist, and a case manager who consistently cared for the cardiac surgery patients. Better working relationships were established with supporting departments, including laboratory, radiology, admissions, and cardiac rehabilitation.

Once these changes were in place, the care environment had a totally different feeling. People enjoyed working together. Patients and families noticed the difference right away. Outcomes immediately improved. Patients were routinely transferred out of the ICU on the first postoperative day, length of stay decreased notably, and deaths and complications became markedly better.

The changes described in these two stories are just a beginning. Additional steps can be taken with staffing, scheduling, and planning to help achieve consistency of interactions in the care environment, with the entire interprofessional team in mind.

Making the familiar effortless, and the unique special

Health care teams care for the same kinds of patients over and over again. Even though each patient is unique, important aspects of care happen in familiar patterns. For example, imagine that today the mother having a baby in our care unit is 30 years old. Her family is with her. Tomorrow she is 15, worried, and alone. The day after that she is 44 and about to deliver the baby she thought she never could have. Each of these women needs care that is familiar (what we do every day), and also care that is special and unique (care just for her).

It might seem that these two kinds of care – care that is familiar and care that is special and unique – could be in conflict. However, our practice and research suggest that successfully providing special care for each person depends on being able to provide familiar care in routine patterns that can become almost effortless. All of this is helped by organizing for teamwork.

If the basic care that a patient needs can become familiar and effortless as a routine, then much more attention can be devoted to the unique care that is special, just for that person.

Summary of things your team can do to organize for teamwork

The care environment can be intentionally organized, staffed, and managed with teamwork in mind. This means that instead of assignments of staff and patients across various settings by role or availability, stable cohorts of people across professions are able to work together as a consistent team in a consistent location, caring for patients with familiarity over time.

- You can intentionally organize your care environment so that the patients you care for are always co-located in a specific area based on their needs and the skills of your team, not randomly sent where space is available.
- You can designate certain areas for certain kinds of care, and small cohorts of specially trained team members for those areas.
- You can put policies in place to assure you can accomplish this – for example, policies that hold beds open so that patients can always be assigned to a specific area.

- You can make staffing and scheduling decisions with the interprofessional team in mind rather than by general assignments across many areas.
- You can organize so that every role on your team is staffed by a designated person or a small group of people who are part of your team – for example, you can be sure that the Pharm D for your team will always be Tom or Sue.
- You can intentionally plan days off and work schedules with the entire team in mind, so that at least 2/3 of the people who here today will work together again tomorrow.
- You can work with leaders of departments that supervise the roles of your team to be sure they understand that staffing and scheduling for a consistent, stable team is a priority over almost any other concern.
- You can intentionally connect with other areas that help to care for your patients – and be proactive about planning and communicating so everyone knows what is coming.
- You can use the times when you are less busy to work on your systems, and train as a team as a high priority, rather than floating people to other areas or sending them home.
- Managers and staff can learn to work from the perspective of having consistent, stable teams– instead of working from the perspective of their own units or departments.

Hard at first to imagine changing like this

When leaders first begin to consider these structural and organizational factors, the challenges of realigning organizational policies and work schedules to create co-location and consistency of interactions may seem overwhelming. Many existing management practices move in the exact opposite direction, such as cross training, admitting to any available bed, floating staff to other areas when the census is low, moving staff and patients out of intensive care to step down areas as acuity changes, etc. In our experience these practices often result in disrupting the relational conditions that collaborative care requires to grow and flourish.

We know from experience that approaches can be found for co-location and consistency, and that care environments structured in these ways will notably outperform those organized in traditional ways. We are not suggesting this is easy. However, anything that can move in this direction will be helpful.

As we have discussed, a foundational precondition for implementing collaborative care is organizing the care environment for consistency of team interactions. If an environment is not structured this way, there will be many practices and expectations that will be difficult or impossible to change, no matter how hard you try.

The good news is that this doesn't have to happen all at once. It is rare that such a major change can be implemented in a single step. A good first step is getting a core group of people together across professions to talk about their work together.

People in organizational leadership positions and also at the front lines need time to consider these changes and try them out in different ways, then gradually adopt them or not, based on their experiences. It may take several years before these kinds of changes make sense to people and can be fully enacted.

The Social Field Model of Collaborative Care accounts for this. Its core elements include the creation of new opportunities for people to meet and talk. Through new interactions and conversations over time, these ideas about different organizing structures can be explored among people and eventually may come to be held differently by them.

On the other hand, if you do have the opportunity to design a care environment from the beginning, you will never regret designing for teamwork from the very first day, carefully matching organizational structures with the natural boundaries of a care team by intentional design. You will not have to take down the old to create the new. It will be much, much easier.

Keeping the Focus on: "What will make this possible?"

If we are asked to help a team implement collaborative care, we encourage the team to take a step back and look at the context in which the new collaborative practices are to be implemented. In our experience, successful implementation of collaborative care requires thoughtful attention to the broader context, and to ways the care environment can be intentionally modified to support the emergence of collaborative care.

A helpful way of doing this is by keeping a clear focus on the question, "What will make this possible?" Asking this question shifts attention upstream, to the preconditions in the care environment that will influence your success.

For everything you hope to accomplish, we encourage you to think and work intentionally upstream, devoting attention to actions and structural changes that make the thing you want to happen become even more likely.

Keep in mind that people do the things they do because those things make sense and have meaning for them. From this perspective you can ask, "What can we change or do differently in our organization and care environment so that collaborative care increasingly makes sense and has greater meaning for people?"

A major lesson of our work is that "people change in conversations." Often it is not the new idea that matters, but how people talk about the new idea. The interventions we advocate focus on creating new structural opportunities for collaborative conversations, where care team members, patients, and family members can interact and converse together in new ways.

Collaborative care comes into being in this generative way, through new structural opportunities that allow new interactions among people, new conversations, and shared reflection together.

The implementation steps of the Social Field Model of Collaborative Care have dual purposes. On the one hand, they create an infrastructure that allows new interactions and conversations that are directly about collaborative care.

Of equal importance, the new interactions and conversations provide opportunities for people to make sense of collaborative care in new ways, with a growing sense of meaning and purpose. We often say that transformation happens at the level of meaning. Once meaning shifts, the rest is easy.

The following sections of the *Field Guide to Collaborative Care* are about activating, deepening, and sustaining collaborative care. In your work and as you read the rest of the Field Guide, ask yourself about your care environment. Do strong preconditions for the emergence and development of collaborative care exist in your care environment? Are there things you can do to make your care environment even more conducive to its emergence?

Keep asking yourself and your team this simple guiding question: What will make this possible?

PART FOUR

ACTIVATING

- Weekly System Meetings
- Daily Collaborative Rounds
- Active Engagement of
  Patients and Families

Weekly System Meetings

In our experience, the most effective way to begin building an exceptional collaborative care environment is by inviting people to participate in weekly system meetings as a new routine. These meetings are your most important implementation intervention.

Establishing a new routine of weekly system meetings creates new opportunities for shared reflection, shared action, and shared learning – setting the stage for the emergence of the contextual resources that make collaborative care possible. We call these meetings "system meetings" because they are about your system of care. Think of these meetings as a way of "making rounds" once a week on your own care team and the systems that support your work together.

We have learned from experience that to be successful at other aspects of collaborative care, such as collaborative rounds, it is invaluable to first create new connections among your team by implementing weekly team meetings. These meetings are not temporary. They are a new element of relational infrastructure in your care environment, a new collaborative home for your team.

Invitations and conversations build connections

People who work together in exceptional collaborative care environments have rich connections. The connections that make exceptional collaborative care possible don't happen by accident. They must be carefully built.

How can you do that? The primary tools for building connections among people are invitations and conversations. That is where to focus your attention. Remember this guiding principle: Collaborative care is built from invitations and conversations.

Collaborative from the beginning

As you think about activating collaborative care, it is helpful to keep in mind some insightful advice about change initiatives:

"*To be successful, the structure of the change initiative must match the structure of the desired final result.*" – Jan Shubert

As applied to implementing collaborative care, this means that the actions that you take as you implement collaborative care should be collaborative from the beginning. The way you begin needs to match your desired goals. You will be most successful if your initial planning group is interprofessional. Collaborative care works best when it is brought into being by people who work well together, are naturally collaborative in their actions, and are respected by their peers.

We have found it especially helpful if a nursing leader and physician leader who work well together are core members of the group of people working to introduce collaborative care. Other health care professionals, patients, and family members can also be very effective as founding members of your initiative.

What is most important is how people work together. The early founding spirit really matters. It will keep showing up again and again as collaborative care grows and develops.

A growing group of interested people

Your team meetings are likely to begin with a small group of people seeking out others who also want to start meeting and working together toward a goal of creating collaborative care.

The figure on the following page shows a small nucleus of people making initial plans, asking for opportunities to meet, having one-on-one conversations, and inviting others to join them.

From these first invitations new connections begin to form, and in a surprisingly short time a growing group of interested people will come together in almost any care environment.

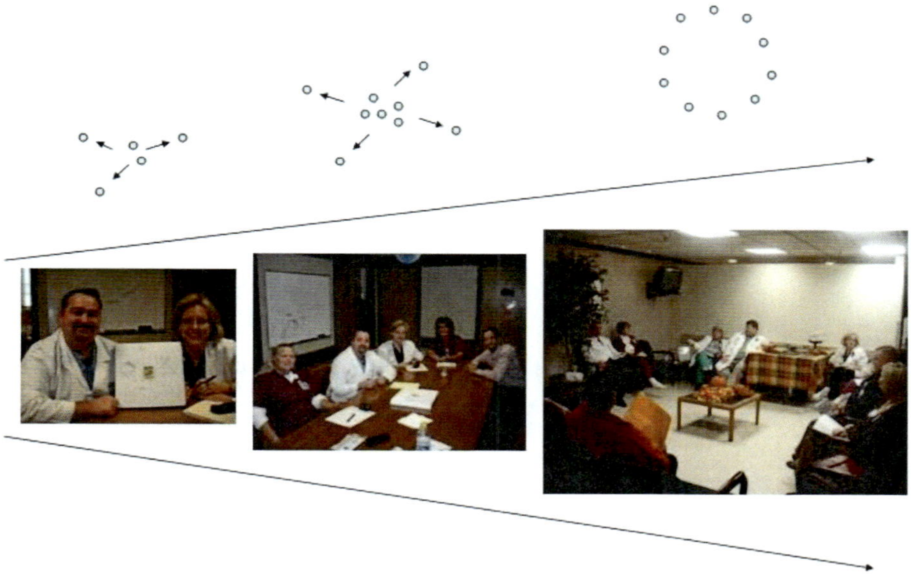

Figure: Actual growth pattern of a new collaborative care initiative:

- **A physician and nurse care manager begin to talk about collaborative care.**
- **They invite other nurses and a pharmacist to meet and talk with them about their hopes and purposes.**
- **Over time others join also, including students and residents. Soon, an inteprofessional group is meeting weekly.**

The panels of the figure show what is likely to happen as you begin. People will be drawn to this work. Your group will grow, evolve, and its nature will shift. The spoke and wheel pattern of early stages will change and soon become a circle.

This progression, from an initiative of one or two people, to a small group of interested people, to a shared effort by an entire team is part of the natural emergence of collaborative care.

In this progressively expanding way, your initial group may decide to extend invitations to people whose participation and support will matter for your initiative. You may also want to offer an open invitation to anyone who might be interested. An open invitation is very important to help avoid the perception that this work is exclusively for a few specially chosen people.

Everything you are doing at this point sets the tone for the collaborative work and is quite symbolic. Be intentionally aware of this. The way you do things at this early stage will show up again and again in the nature and spirit of what you do later. You are forming the culture of your collaborative team with every action, and especially so in these early stages

Envisioning and inviting your team

It is helpful to imagine what you hope your collaborative care environment will be like, and to base your initial invitations on that picture. The Collaborative Care TEAMFINDER can be helpful for this. We suggest that you consider using this tool at an early stage to help your team envision the roles and connections you need to be at your best, then inviting those people.

There will be people whom it will seem natural to invite, either because of the roles they have or their individual strengths. There will also be some people you might imagine would never want to be involved. You will be surprised, though, as you begin to invite people.

We suggest not having too many preconceptions. In our experience you will be surprised who turns out to be interested and who will make contributions. If you decide not to invite someone, it will be noticed. It is almost always wiser to err on the side of inclusion. Again, remember you are establishing the culture of your collaborative initiative by the actions you are taking.

Meetings are the heartbeat of your team

A helpful agreement for getting people to come is to make it clear that they are not required to attend, and that you know they are busy and may not be able to stay for the full meeting. They are welcome to attend if they can.

We encourage you to invite people to come when they can, and to catch up when they can't. Make an agreement that it is OK for people to come late or leave early if necessary. That is the nature of health care. Make it comfortable for people to attend, even if only for a short time.

It is vital for your success to develop a routine of having consistent meetings. Set a pattern that people can count on. Think of the meetings as the heartbeat of your team. We have found that it is important to have a schedule and keep to it, no matter who can or can't attend. Even if only a few people are able to be there on a particular day, and especially if a particular leader can't come, have the meeting right on time anyway.

Remember that your team can change its mind about when and where to meet. Many teams move the time and place of their weekly meeting once or twice until they find the right time and place that works for most people.

The first goal is simply to keep meeting

Your first goal at first is simply to leave each meeting with an agreement to have additional meetings! The meetings should be held at a convenient time and place so that people can attend while still caring for their patients. Make sure that people are able to sit facing one another, close enough so they can talk easily.

Welcome people and thank them for coming. Take time to listen about everyone's interest in collaborative care and invite people to talk about their reasons for being present. Be thoughtful about establishing a respectful, welcoming environment where people feel comfortable and valued.

There will probably be a question at this point about how often your team should meet. People will feel very busy and will not be sure they can take the time to attend if the meetings are held too frequently.

Take advantage of this question as an opportunity to practice making room in your conversations for these differences, for "holding" different viewpoints and still being functional as a team. As you do, this ability will grow.

We recommend having these meetings every week if at all possible, as an ongoing new routine that is intended to become part of your normal work. If meetings occur less frequently, too much will happen during the intervening days, and the real work will shift outside of these meetings into other sites and settings.

Food is helpful

Food helps! It is easier to attract people to your meeting when they know they will be able to eat something. Also, it is hard to sit down and eat together while holding on to hierarchy.

In our experience, planning for some sort of food for your meetings really makes a difference. It can be lunch, some special treat that someone makes or brings, or even chocolate. Yummy!

Careful attention to connections with the larger organization

As you begin to establish your collaborative system meetings, remember to ask for the advice and support of organizational leaders interested and responsible for what you plan to accomplish. This is important no matter where you are positioned in the organization, even if you are a very senior leader and everyone reports to you.

Collaborative care will probably be a significant change from usual ways of working in your organization, a more significant change than even at first it might seem. It asks different things and requires different strengths of managers and leaders than most are familiar with in traditional health care.

Careful attention to informing, inviting, and engaging people is helpful and wise for increasing chances of success and preventing surprises and difficulties at later stages of this work.

Others will notice and have their own stories to tell about what you are doing. Help them understand what you are doing by including them, and ask for their advice about how to align this work with the mission and goals that matter to them.

How to run the meetings

One of the interesting decisions you will make together about the meetings is how they will be run. Our suggestion is to keep the meetings relatively informal. We also suggest that you talk among yourselves about who should moderate or lead the meetings. There may be an expectation that formal leaders should lead the meetings. If so, the meetings will tend to be like other meetings people are used to having.

We suggest that you change that traditional expectation to something more comfortable and participatory. One way to do that is by inviting people from middle levels of the usual hierarchy to lead the meetings. There will probably be several people who are interested and will be ideal for this role. The meetings will feel different, more participatory and generative, when this kind of non-traditional hierarchy leadership is adopted.

The role of formal leaders regarding these meetings is interesting. In our experience the optimum role for formal leaders is that of engaged participant. All eyes will be on the formal leader, especially when differences arise and when decisions and plans are being made. It is important for formal leaders to be self-aware about this, and to use these moments to demonstrate in their actions respect and confidence in the wisdom and abilities of the entire team.

It is easy to fall into a pattern of leaders deciding and directing. It takes sensitivity and patience for formal leaders to step back and let the group lead, converse, and decide together.

Appreciating a different kind of power

Utilizing the team meetings for discussions and collective decision making lets people learn about and try out a surprising kind of power, made possible to leaders by inviting participation rather than by deciding and directing.

One of the most significant shifts in collaborative care is the leadership role of traditional leaders, including physicians. It is extremely rewarding for leaders to lead in a collaborative, participatory way rather than the more traditional role of deciding and directing. However, it may not be easy for leaders to know this at first, when first experiencing collaborative care. The team meetings are a way of letting people try leading like this. Most leaders will find this rewarding, although some will not like it at all.

As your team engages in collaborative leadership, you will notice that the team's sense of identity strengthens, and that your understanding of leadership will begin to change. All of this requires time and opportunities to try this out and become familiar and comfortable with these new ways of interacting together. The team meetings can become a safe and respectful place to work these things out, away from the stresses of direct patient care.

A short agenda with plenty of white space

An interesting conversation will be about an agenda for the meetings. We have observed there is usually a difference in comfort among people about this. Some people will enjoy an open and unstructured chance to talk about anything that comes up, and other people will want a clearly specified agenda.

We have found that a middle ground of a short regular agenda with plenty of white space for open discussion is a good balance that keeps most people happy and engaged. At some point in the meeting a "round table" discussion format that gives a structured opportunity for each person to make a contribution or ask a question can be very helpful in expanding participation.

This pattern of "going around the circle" gives people a chance for contributing thoughts that might otherwise never be said. By taking these intentional actions you are making sure that the environment you are creating is inviting and welcoming of new people and their contributions. Again, these actions are establishing the culture of your team that will show up in many ways later, including on collaborative rounds.

Intentionally creating a safe place for many viewpoints

As people become comfortable enough to talk about their concerns or worries, be sure this is acknowledged and valued. You want people to be able to express concerns in the meetings, because if not, these concerns will still be talked about, but in other conversations where people can't respond as a group.

Work hard to become comfortable with the ambiguity and uncertainty that is always a part of collaboration. Remember that collaboration does not mean consensus or uniformity.

People will notice and come

Once there starts to be a buzz about the weekly meeting as a place to bring and resolve ideas and to discuss possibilities, more people will start to attend. If people can be sure the meeting will happen every week, and that their ideas and concerns will be respectfully considered, they will bring their thoughts and hopes.

Doing things that matter

People will accept invitations and will begin to participate in response to invitations and curiosity. But curiosity will only keep them coming for at most three or four meetings.

For people to continue to come, prioritizing these meetings over the endless other ways they could spend their time and invest their energies, there must be some satisfaction that makes participation meaningful to them.

If people are able to see that they can truly participate, and find that their participation makes some kind of a difference, it is very likely they will continue to come. Keep this thought in mind in your early meetings and find ways to assure that the meetings matter. Let people see that the meeting accomplishes things.

One way of making an impact is by having decision makers present so that changes can be made on the spot rather than making recommendations and waiting. Increasingly, try to make these meetings the place where major decisions about your care environment are discussed and made.

It may seem that meeting and talking are activities that take time away from patient care, something nice to do but not your real work. One of the most important insights of the Social Field Model is that some of the most important work happening in your care environment happens in these meetings.

As will be described in greater detail later, the special capabilities of reliability and resilience are created through action and reflection at a group level. When you look at these meetings, try to envision what is being made in them as people meet and talk together. Reliability and resilience are being created here.

New routines will build a new culture

As these meetings are first forming, your team is establishing routines together that, once formed, you will see again and again in many other kinds of activities later on. You are developing your team culture with the patterns you set.

One very helpful pattern that will bring great returns later is establishing a routine of starting each meeting with introductions and welcoming everyone. This is helpful even if people have worked together for a long time. It is often the case that people don't know one another by name, even though they may have worked together for years.

A pattern of introductions and welcoming as a normal routine can help overcome those awkward moments when we know we should know someone but we don't. It is a small thing to do that helps to build richer connections. If people aren't quite sure of a person's name, they may act in a way that shields them from any kind of interaction that would reveal what they don't know. By making it easy for people to know everyone's name as a routine, interactions often become more comfortable for people.

It is particularly useful to invite people to introduce themselves by asking something that goes beyond a simple statement of name or role. You will be surprised by what you learn about each other, and how this new knowledge changes how your team works together. You will be surprised what you learn about the people you have worked with for a long time that you did not know. You will also be interested in what you learn about the other professions you work with. You will see the value of this in your work. Things will come up that you have discussed. You will notice things you didn't see before.

As this happens, talk about it with your team in your meetings. Encourage and model becoming comfortable reflecting together about these growing insights, with appreciation. Again, you are establishing patterns that will show up later. You will appreciate having a comfortable pattern of introductions and welcoming, and reflecting together about new insights, as your team progresses to other activities such as collaborative rounds.

Also, it is very helpful to make a point of warmly welcoming people who come late, and of acknowledging and thanking people who have to leave early. Although people may want to sneak in and out quietly, it is helpful to develop a routine of welcoming people when they arrive and thanking people when they leave. Every person who comes or goes changes the room in some way. Your meetings will function even better if comings and goings are acknowledged and contributions are intentionally appreciated.

These actions can be introduced intentionally by members of the group early on, and are likely to become group norms. It is through these early intentional steps and their repetition over time – and the experiences and feelings that these patterns begin to make possible – that a collaborative social field is constructed.

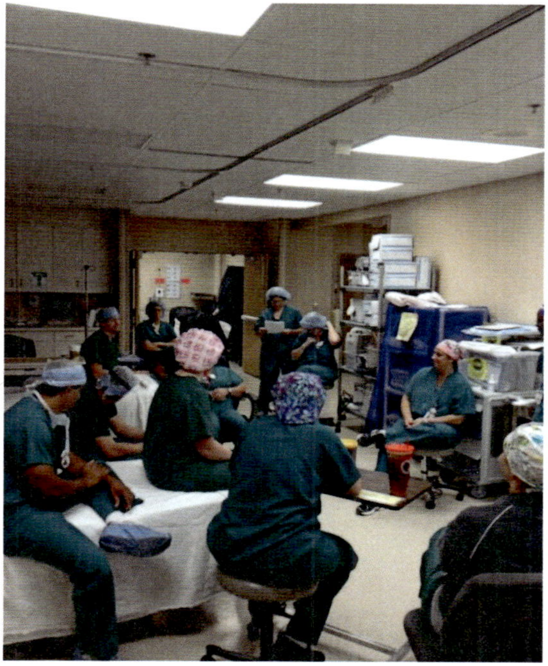

Photo: Weekly System Meeting, OR Team

In time, these weekly meetings will become the central home for the work of building your collaborative care processes.

The weekly system meetings give people a chance to talk and reflect together away from the stress of active patient care, and get to know one another in new and richer ways as people as well as in their professional roles.

At first in our research, we did not realize how important these weekly meetings are. Over time, we came to realize that they are a major infrastructure element needed for success. All other activities build upon and are brought back to this meeting.

The primary place where decisions are made

We strongly encourage leaders and other team members to utilize the weekly team meetings as the primary place where possibilities are discussed and all major decisions are made.

If this is intentionally done, the meetings will become the central home for the leadership, values, beliefs, and meaning that guide the practices of the collaborative program.

At first, this may be hard for traditional leaders. It is a departure from usual routines in health care, where leaders often ask others for input but then make decisions on their own, and concerns are often viewed as best handled privately and behind closed doors. It takes intentional effort to shift these established routines toward an open, collaborative approach.

A basic goal and principle is that everything that happens in the care environment that affects the team should be brought to these meetings. An early emphasis on team-level reflection and decision making with shared planning and monitoring will establish a pattern that can be built upon and expanded later.

This collective way of talking together and making decisions together is likely to seem puzzling at first for many people, especially those not part of the meetings. People will want to bring concerns to leaders in private settings as they have always done. Leaders can significantly help the development of the team meetings by asking that people "save" conversations until everyone can be present. This, too, will seem puzzling at first until the value of the collaborative conversations becomes clear.

Gradually, as your team is able to establish new norms around this, people will begin to see that the insights and responses made possible in the meetings are surprisingly effective and unexpectedly satisfying. Understanding and appreciation for collaborative discussions and decision making will grow as people gain firsthand experience working this way.

Regular meetings are a show of commitment and a key element of the infrastructure of collaborative care. Being able to count on having a meeting together every week is helpful as the team moves through the work of implementing other collaborative activities, including collaborative rounds. Consistency will also draw those whose tendency is to "wait and see". You may want to take time in an early meeting to use suggestions from the *Collaborative Care Activation Inventory (CCAI)* as a guide for ways to make these weekly meetings even better.

As will be discussed, the weekly team meetings are an important relational platform that supports team learning. The team meetings are the "Reflection" half of the action-reflection cycles described in later sections, and are essential for achieving reliability and resilience. The weekly meeting becomes the place where your team asks and answers the questions: How are we doing together as a team? What can we do even better?

Inviting patients and family members from the outset

One question worth considering is whether to invite patients and families to be part of these initial team meetings as you first begin. Your team probably knows patients and family members that you could invite to your system meetings who would be valuable in helping to create your collaborative care environment.

Our advice is twofold about patient and family engagement at an early stage. First, if you are able to engage patients and families from the beginning, you will be miles ahead. Second, in our experience it seems to be difficult for many teams to open themselves at an early stage to engagement with patients and families in this way.

A feeling of needing to "get our own house in order" before inviting patients and families into this work is often strong. Over time this will change, and involving patients and families will become much more comfortable. However, at first it may be perceived as too stressful.

You may find it helpful to use the *Collaborative Care Activation Inventory (CCAI)* to explore ideas about patient and family engagement in your system meetings and see what people say. You will know what is best. Do it if you can.

A new understanding of meetings

Often in health care most meetings are thought of as a waste of time, or at best a necessary evil. Stop and reflect about what those dreaded meetings are like. They are often run from a heavy agenda, and are often a way of pushing information and decisions that have already been made.

In contrast, the weekly system meetings we are advocating are intended to be a forum for ideas and reflection linked with action from all levels of the care team. With this clearly in view from the beginning, you will create a very different kind of meeting, one that has a new kind of reward and meaning for people.

Some teams call these meetings "System Rounds." One team leader said, "We make rounds on our patients every day, and once a week we make rounds on our systems of care." The leader continued, "That is what those meetings are for. They are a place we can look thoughtfully at ourselves and what we are doing, and imagine how we might do even better."

It has been remarkable to us as researchers how much these meetings are appreciated and continue to be well attended over the long run, despite how busy people are. They seem to meet some sort of human need for connecting with others. They become a place to meet, talk, get to know one another in new ways, and maintain perspective on what is being done and why. Even when other parts of a collaborative initiative are struggling, the weekly team meetings seem to survive.

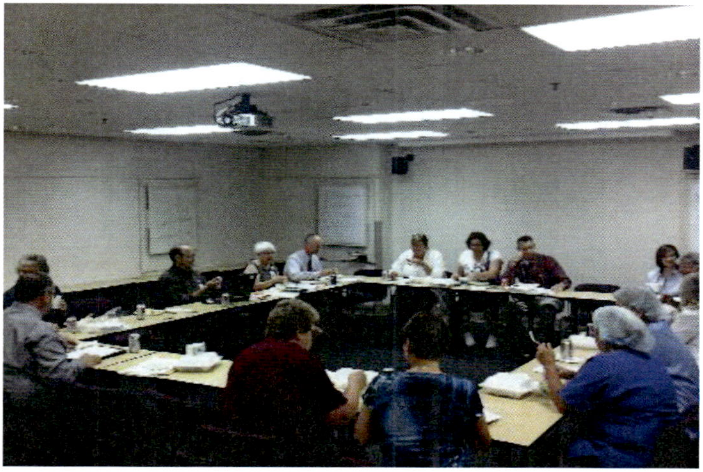

Photo: Weekly System Meeting, Wesley Medical Center, Wichita, Kansas

The photo above shows a weekly meeting of a care team at Wesley Medical Center in Wichita, Kansas. These meetings have happened every Tuesday at noon since 2009.

Devoting attention to developing the social field

If you are reading this book, you are probably interested in implementing interprofessional collaborative rounds with active engagement of patients and families. We are very interested in this, too, and a following section is written to help your team implement this essential daily activity of collaborative care.

However, we strongly suggest from theory and experience that you be patient and wait before beginning daily collaborative rounds until your care team has been meeting regularly as a collaborative team for a period of time.

Why wait? Collaborative rounds is a significant relational accomplishment that is achieved and appreciated through experience over time. The more we have learned about collaborative care, the more we recognize that weekly system meetings are essential for the success of daily collaborative rounds and other collaborative care activities.

Weekly system meetings and daily collaborative rounds are interrelated parts of the social field of a collaborative team. In other words, we have come to understand that collaborative rounds is affected by many things outside of rounds itself. It was startling and humbling to us that we could not see this at first.

To be successful at implementing collaborative care, it is necessary to devote attention to making intentional structural and relational changes in your care environment – strengthening relational infrastructure to develop your social field.

By waiting to begin daily collaborative rounds until after weekly team meetings are well established, you will have developed many important new connections in your developing social field, and will have a comfortable place and new routines for reflecting on your work together outside of the stress of daily patient care. We have found this is very important for success.

A spirit of trying

As you develop the routines of your team meetings, one thing to keep in mind is that you are setting new norms that will shape what it is like to work in your care environment.

In general, we encourage teams to develop and model a "spirit of trying." This means intentionally becoming comfortable trying new things, always with an awareness of the comfort boundaries of your team, yet in ways that intentionally encourage the team to explore and progressively expand the limits of those boundaries. One person said, "We won't know until we try."

By establishing a "spirit of trying" as a norm of your team, you are intentionally laying foundations for the later growth and development of team level capabilities for being comfortable exploring new approaches that are necessary for resilience. You are also helping to establish a context that will support the growth of reliability and responsiveness.

Summary of things your team can do to establish weekly meetings

Structures and routines for collective reflection can be intentionally established – for example, weekly system meetings to review and improve how the team works together. Having these structures and routines provides a place to develop additional connections and understandings across roles, and to monitor, discuss and improve systems and processes for working together.

- You can meet as a team every week to reflect about your work together – these meetings aren't about patient care, they are to reflect together about how you work as a team.

- Make these meetings the primary place for discussing anything that involves your unit – do this so everyone can be aware and involved.

- Remember to keep the spirit of the meeting open and informal even though it is an important meeting – you want this to be inviting and interesting and not a burden for people.

- Make it a routine to invite other departments and people to join the meetings, especially when you talk about things that involve them so you can listen and include them.

- Even though formal leaders are present and participating, rotate who runs the meeting so it doesn't feel like meetings in which people are being told what to do.

- Bring food to the meetings – it gets people to come and it seems easier to work together across roles and with a more level hierarchy when you are eating together.

- Reflect on how much you may not know about one another even though many of you have worked together for years – use the meetings as a time to see each other in new ways.

- Maintain a pattern of introducing yourselves around the table even when no one new is present – it helps everyone get to know one another and creates a pattern of participation.

- Use a short agenda for each meeting with a lot of white space for new concerns or suggestions – this is a good balance that seems to meet most people's expectations.

- Make sure decision makers with authority attend the meetings so you can decide in the meeting to do doing things differently without having to wait for approval elsewhere.

Daily Collaborative Rounds

We have watched daily collaborative rounds begin in many ways. Often people will just want to get on with it. Although we advise against this, don't worry if your team wants to just jump right in. Your team needs to learn for itself how to do this. Go ahead and start if people want to, and remember that you can come back to what is written here if you need additional guidance.

As your team is forming and developing, at some point you will be ready to begin planning for collaborative rounds. There is no "right time" to begin, just know that it will take a while to be ready for this in a way that is successful and sustainable. Remember that collaborative care takes time to grow and develop. Your team is more likely to succeed with collaborative rounds if your approach is gradual, thoughtful, and incremental.

Planning for daily collaborative rounds

Most people need to think about their work in new ways before collaborative rounds will become meaningful for them. These new ways of understanding are arrived at through conversations, reflections, and having new experiences together.

To be successful, you will want to invite many people to help plan the new care process. Your efforts will go backwards if you tell people that, as of today, we will now make collaborative rounds. Collaborative care is built with invitations, not directives.

Remember that the actions taken as your team prepares for collaborative rounds are establishing a new culture. The way you do things at first will show up later in what your rounds will eventually be like. You are establishing the "heart and soul" of your rounds by the way you approach things as you first begin.

Your team will need to consider many things as you prepare for collaborative rounds, including what rounds will be like, who will be involved, when the rounds will happen, where the rounds will be held, and how you will engage your team, patients, and family members. Keep in mind that your rounds will evolve and improve as you gain experience working collaboratively.

Consider beginning with simulations

In our experience, a really good way of working out how to do collaborative rounds is to begin with simulations. Also, keep in mind that you can come back to simulations if your first efforts don't go well. Many teams have found this to be helpful.

Simulation of collaborative rounds doesn't require any special equipment. All it requires is a spare patient room, a few interested people, and a little time.

Choose a day and a reasonable amount of time, perhaps an hour, that is enough so you can try some things but won't feel too burdensome for people. Have a person act in the role of the patient, and another person or two can be family members. Imagine a clinical situation you often see, and use an empty room to practice making rounds together.

Here are some things you might practice:

Practice foaming your hands and walking into the patient's room. What if you need gowns and gloves? Where will people stand? Should anyone sit down? Who will talk first? How will you introduce yourselves to the patient and family? Can you do this in a way that invites people to participate? Practice inviting the patient and family to join your circle, and ask them to participate in introductions. Ask your patient and family participants how it felt to participate in these ways, and what would be ideal for them.

Try to go through an entire rounds flow. See if you can remember to talk with the patient and family in ordinary language. Listen to the language you are using. Can an ordinary person understand what is being said?

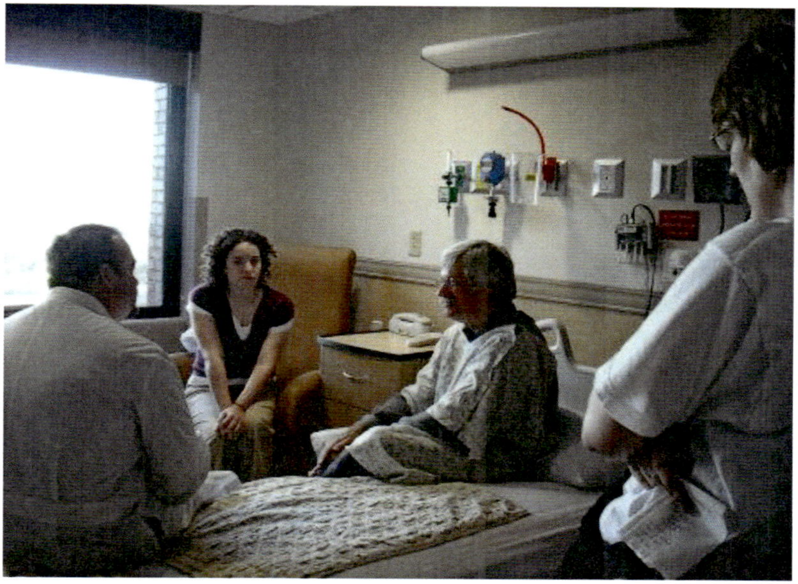

Photo: Simulation of Collaborative Rounds with patient/family actors

Take a minute and note how you are sitting or standing, and who is talking with whom. Is someone sitting at eye level with the patient? Are you keeping your circle open to the patient and family, including them in what is happening, or have you closed your circle to them? Are you looking at and talking directly with the patient and family, or has your team lapsed into talking to each other in medical language again?

Practice asking the patient and family about life outside of the hospital – for example, where the patient lives and what he or she enjoys doing. See if you can incorporate that knowledge about the patient into your conversations about the medical care.

Discuss the things you need to do medically for the patient, and who will get those things accomplished during rounds. Ask your patient and family representatives if they feel included. Are their needs, thoughts, and concerns being heard?

Try talking about things that aren't going well, or about mistakes or errors that may have happened. Try out what you might say. Is it comfortable having these conversations with patients and family members? Or is it your instinct to wait to discuss these things outside the room? See what it is like if you open those conversations to everyone. Ask people what it felt like to talk about mistakes. You may be surprised what you learn.

Practice what you will do differently on the second day or third day compared to the first. Did the second day take less time? Practice what you will do when new members of your team come who are unfamiliar with the rounds process. How will you guide them so they feel included and comfortable right away?

Moving from simulations to actual patient care

At some point, your team will be ready to begin actual collaborative patient care. We suggest that when your team feels ready, thoughtfully select a patient who needs straightforward care and ask for permission from that patient to try collaborative rounds with them and their family members.

Tell the patient what you are doing and how much it will help your team to do this. Then recall what you have practiced and learned in simulations and try the real thing.

As part of your rounds, take a moment and ask your patient and family members what their experience of rounds is like. You will be surprised how much they know and notice. You will probably see that your relationship with that patient and family is different already, just from this.

Ask other team members what they noticed. Ask what rounds was like for everyone present, including the patient and family. What people see and what you learn will surprise you.

The next day, try it again. When you do so, invite your patient and family to help you make your rounds even better.

Gradually, take on more complex patients and try seeing more patients collaboratively. Start with one patient a day, then two. At some point make a commitment to caring for all patients this way as your new normal routine. That will take a while.

Stay within comfort limits of time, and recognize that it will take more time to provide care this way at first. As you talk about care and time, consider the time it takes to see the patients, and also consider time people save later by what you are able to accomplish. For most people, collaborative care saves more time than it adds, and people will recognize the care is a lot better. But it takes a while for that awareness to develop.

Especially as you are beginning, there will be days and moments when people are too stressed by events to take the time needed for collaborative care. We suggest on those days to respect this discomfort and let people do what makes sense to them at the time. Then come back the next day and start again.

Eventually, you will be able to make collaborative rounds for every patient. However, for all the reasons above, we suggest that you start slowly at first and work steadily toward this goal. Keep trying and keep learning, always going back and forth between the action of care and reflection about care. See patients together, talk and reflect together, consider what you can do even better or differently, then try again. That is the learning cycle.

Your team will figure out over time what works for you. In our experience, it will take six to eight months for new collaborative care routines to become fully established in your care environment. There will be ups and downs and several re-beginnings before lasting success.

Secrets of success

In the next parts of this section we will talk about some interesting nuances that your team will experience as you develop collaborative rounds. We have found that there are specific actions that can be helpful as a care team develops collaborative rounds. The following suggestions may be useful as your care team navigates this together. Remember, there is no single way that is "right." You will develop your own methods and patterns that work well in your own care environment.

The ability to invite and welcome

One of the most important capabilities of a collaborative care team is the ability to invite and welcome others into this way of working together. This is true for professional members of the team welcoming other professional members, and is especially true as the professional care team opens itself with warmth and invitation to patients and families.

The invitation and welcoming into the bedside rounds process begins outside the room as the team is assembling. We believe every effort should be made to avoid a somewhat natural tendency to begin talking about the patient's condition among the team outside of a context where the patient and family can participate. This commitment to including the patient and family in every conversation and interaction is an intentional leadership action that can be taken by all members of the team and can be reinforced with phrases such as, "nothing about me without me."

Inviting and welcoming continues as the team enters the room and begins to establish connections with the patient and family through eye contact, greetings, and specific invitations for the patient and family to join the rounds process. This includes invitations and reassurances that participation of the patient and family in rounds is very important and very welcome.

Inviting and welcoming includes nonverbal actions such as one or more members of the team sitting at eye level with the patient and family, and intentional pacing of speech, cadence, listening, and attentiveness that communicate a commitment and willingness to take time to fully engage at levels that go beyond attention to technical and medical details.

Start with introductions

We suggest beginning rounds by going around the circle with brief introductions by name and professional role. This simple routine is remarkably effective in creating an expectation of inclusion and participation by everyone present.

This includes verbal and nonverbal gestures that invite and gently guide the patient and family members to include themselves in the introduction process. It is helpful if one or more members of the professional care team offers a short introductory description to the rounds process and its purpose. An example for introducing rounds might be saying something like,

"Good morning, Mr. Smith. This is our daily collaborative care rounds. We are glad to see you and delighted your family is here. Our purpose is to be sure that we are all on the same page,

and that all of us, including you and your family, are working together to take the best, safest, care of you possible."

We have been fascinated by how these small rituals make such a big difference in how the rounds is perceived by patients and families. They only take a few seconds, yet the room feels very different after you have made these initial welcoming actions.

Talk "with" patients, not "about" them

Throughout all of these activities, every effort should be made to talk directly with the patient and family members as the primary conversation, and to intentionally avoid discussions exclusively between care team members whenever possible.

Medical conversations may be necessary at points in the rounds. However, even during these times every effort should be made to include the patient and family members in what is being said. This can be done by using ordinary language and being intentionally aware of non-verbal body language.

Try to be sure that all of the interactions on rounds indicate inclusion and welcoming, and avoid signaling that the team is having a separate conversation from which the patient is excluded.

Use of a goal board

One of the things you can practice is using a goal board. As plans are developed, it is quite useful to record the plans on a goal board in the patient's room. The goal board is a shared conceptual space that allows the entire care team, including the patient and family members, to track and contribute to the emerging plan. The goal board serves as a reminder and memory device that holds the care plans for all to see until the next bedside meeting.

In many care environments we have visited, there are often standardized white boards in patient rooms with formatted spaces for information. In general, we have found that white boards formatted like this are not very useful for collaborative care. We have found that simpler is better when it comes to the format of the goal board. Some teams just use pieces of poster paper stuck to the wall. It is important to have a space large enough to write many goals every day, in writing big enough for everyone, including the patient and family, to read easily.

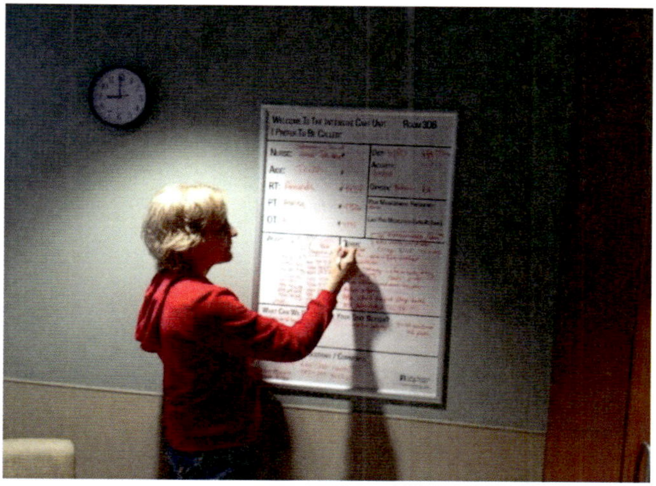

Photo: The daughter of a patient updating the goal board. This became her daily role during collaborative rounds.

In highly developed collaborative care, maintaining the goal board during rounds may become the responsibility of a family member. It can also be very useful for students, who write and summarize on the board as part of their learning experience. Are there HIPAA concerns about a goal board? Simply ask your patient if it is OK. With permission, using the goal board is fine.

We encourage writing items down on the goal board that are personal for the patient. Write comments in the patient's own words. Goals such as, "Go home soon but not too soon," or "likes spaghetti and tomatoes but not chocolate pudding" alongside "CT scan today" and "Recheck K 3.2" are powerful connections with the life of the person being cared for.

A systematic review of the goal board is a powerful closing action for the team, patient, and family at the end of each day's rounds, recapping goals and clarifying responsibilities. An opening review of the board the next day carries the entire team back in time, helping everyone remember the information, circumstances, emotions, and plans that were jointly developed and experienced. Erasing items from the goal board as they are accomplished and watching the goal list change day-by-day is a way of keeping aligned together with a shared sense of progress.

In our observations, the way the goal board is used is a marker of the acceptance of the collaborative rounds process. In early stages a few people may refer to the goal board, but often others don't. Over time, the team is likely to devote greater attention to the goal board, referring to it and using it throughout the day for things like shift to shift handovers. Families often refer to the goal board with other family members who were not present for rounds, bringing them up to date about what is happening.

Use of a safety checklist

One of the most helpful ways of assuring reliability is incorporating the use of a checklist into your daily care. The checklist can be developed by your team to include things that you want to be sure to double check every day, for every patient.

Finding the right balance about what to include on the checklist will take a little testing. Putting too many things on the checklist will frustrate people, yet having a daily reminder of key things will make it much more likely that you won't miss anything. An example of a safety checklist developed by a cardiac surgery team is shown on the next page. Your team may want to emphasize different things. It is not the checklist that matters, but developing it and using it together that makes the difference.

Daily Rounds Safety Checklist

- Blood Clot Prevention?
- Blood Sugar Control?
- Lines and Tubes?
- Skin and Wounds?
- Aspirin, Statin, B Blocker, ACEI?
- Home Medications?
- Nutrition?
- Fall Risk?

Figure: Example of a safety checklist for daily care

Take time to include patients and families as you go over the checklist. Run down the list point by point, and invite everyone to consider each item. Patients will appreciate being included in this and will watch these things closely with you. Practice the use of a checklist for things you want to be sure you do every time. Talk about what should be on the checklist and how you will use it.

An intentional shift from individual to collective work

An important point should be made here regarding participation of various professional members of the health care team, and participation of patients and family members. This concerns a shift of mindset from individual participation to collective participation. There is often a tendency early in the development of the rounds process for individual team members to continue to approach this work from an individual perspective rather than envisioning their work as part of a collective effort.

A major area of growth that requires early attention is creating an expectation that each person present will remain attentive and will actively participate, listening and maintaining interest and engagement during the entire rounds conversation, being a part of the shared conversation that is happening among all team members and with patients and families.

Early, as collaborative care is being introduced, we have frequently seen professional care team members continue other tasks during rounds, such as scanning the patient's wristband, checking IV fluids, and even sticking a patient's finger to check blood glucose as the rounds conversation is happening.

Usually when this happens, it is an indication that people are not yet "seeing" the rounds differently. Some people who have shifted to a collective orientation will be looking with amazement that such actions could happen, whereas others will not give this a thought, because it makes perfect sense to them from the more traditional perspective of individual work that needs to be done.

Another indicator of active engagement is whether people have side conversations with one another, turn away from the collective circle when they are not talking, gather data from a chart or from the computer, or pursue other individual actions.

It is easy at first for people to believe their attention or contribution is not needed at certain points because of the topic being discussed. Respectful redirection may be needed here to remind people to stay engaged and attentive, and to help create a shared conversation among everyone present. This is a definite change from usual patterns and may take some time to develop.

There is a risk that people may feel criticized by this redirection, yet it can usually be done. One approach is taking a moment as a team to reflect on the goal of creating a shared conversation space, and that to be respectful as a team this needs to be established. Redirections are usually received in a receptive way if they are made respectfully.

This can be as simple as just always going around the circle and asking each person to say something. Rounds will be much richer as your team becomes comfortable allowing the pattern of the rounds process to initiate who speaks, rather than prompts or questions from a leader who is asking or directing.

Related to this is an expectation that each person will make active contributions. In early stages there is often a tendency for people to say, "I have nothing to add." It is helpful if everyone knows that each person will be given an opportunity to actively participate, and that this is a shared expectation.

Developing a comfortable pattern

With practice and experience, your team will figure out a stable pattern for collaborative rounds that works well in your care environment.

The main principle is having a rounds conversation that includes and engages everyone present, and gives equal opportunity for everyone to make observations, ask questions, and contribute to the assessment and plan.

A guide for daily collaborative rounds used by several teams is shown on the following pages.

Daily Collaborative Rounds Guide

- **Introductions**

After coming into the room, everyone assembles in a circle around the patient's bed. The patient is greeted and family members are welcomed and invited to join the circle.

All who are present introduce themselves around the circle by name and role. Family members and the patient are invited to introduce themselves along with the professional care team members.

The conversation is intentionally kept mostly in ordinary language and is directed to the patient and family who are included as essential participants.

- **Welcoming and purpose of rounds**

"Good morning, Mr. Smith. This is our daily collaborative care rounds. We are glad to see you and delighted your family is here. Our purpose is to be sure that we are all on the same page, and that all of us, including you and your family, are working together to take the best, safest, care of you possible."

- **Learning something about the patient as a person**

"Before we talk about the medical details of your care, we would like to take a minute to learn more about you as a person. Would you mind telling us something about yourself, for example, where you live, or things that you especially enjoy doing?"

Make brief notes on the Goal Board of special interests and first names and relationships of family members. Sometimes a drawing is useful, for example, of golf clubs.

You will find it helpful to glance at these reminders each day during rounds. They will help everyone remember about the patient as a person and what matters to him/her.

- **Bedside nurse update and review of yesterday's goal board**

  This is spoken in ordinary language to the patient with the rest of the team following along, not a typical report to the care team in medical language.

  Complete medical and technical details are included and are translated or explained as necessary.

- **"Around the Circle" starting with the patient and family**

  "Mr. Smith, we are going to go around our circle to talk about your care together, starting with you. Do you have any questions, suggestions, goals or concerns today?"

  Each person around the circle then has an opportunity to add thoughts, questions, and recommendations to an evolving group discussion of assessment and planning.

  As things come up that matter or action items arise, they are written on the Goal Board. Some goals are in the patient's own words, "Home soon but not too soon;" others are medical, "Pulmonary consult," "Watch creatinine (2.1)."

- **Safety Checklist**

  Systematically review essential safety items for every patient using a safety checklist the team has developed.

- **GLITCH – Could anything have been different or better?**

  Pause to ask the patient, family and other team members if anything could have been different or better in the last 24 hours. "GLITCHes" (see pp. 177-184) are listened and responded to, and recorded for the weekly system meeting.

- **Recap and review of Goal Board**

  Recap what is planned and who will do what.

- **Anything else?**

  Make a final check around the circle that everyone is OK.

Meet and reflect as a team every day

As you make the transition to actual bedside collaborative care, one of the most helpful things you can do is to establish a daily reflective session, maybe 30 minutes each afternoon, as part of your new daily routines. These sessions provide your team with opportunities to reflect and debrief about the work you are doing to implement daily collaborative rounds.

Meghan Crabtree is a research graduate student who made detailed observations during implementation of daily collaborative rounds on a hospital medicine teaching service. The care team she observed made collaborative rounds each morning, and came together again at 1:30 each afternoon to reflect about their progress. Meghan could see important changes happening during the daily reflective sessions over the month that she observed the work of the team. She concluded that the daily reflective sessions allowed the team to:

-reflect on the day's successes and stumbling blocks

-plan for the next day's activities

-make incremental changes to the rounds routines

-communicate plans and ideas across disciplines

-follow up with others on specific patient discussions

-develop and strengthen relationships

-decompress

It was not an easy change for the team that she observed to go from traditional rounds to collaborative rounds. Meghan felt that the daily reflective sessions were important for the team's success. Meghan documented the conversations that occurred in the reflective meetings and showed how the conversations changed over time. During the first week, the conversations were usually about how hard things were. Over the next several weeks the conversations changed and became more hopeful. By the end of the first month, the conversations had shifted and now focused on what else was needed to keep the rounds going.

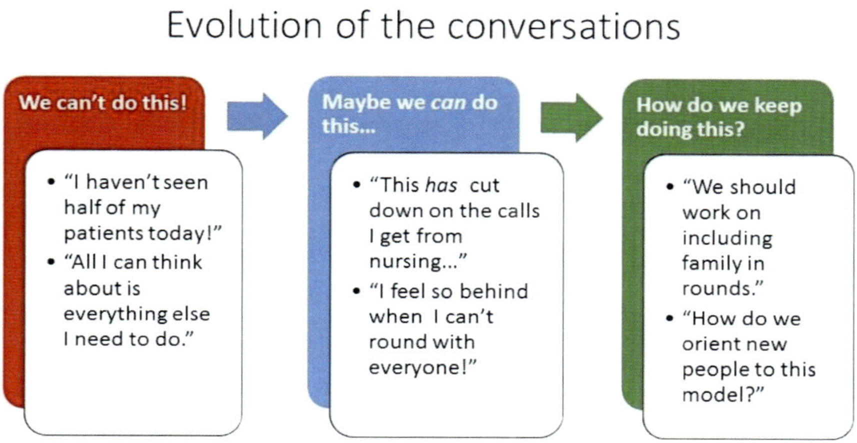

Figure: Evolution in daily reflective sessions (Meghan Crabtree)

The daily reflection sessions are intended to take place in addition to the weekly team meetings described in the preceding section. The two reflective meetings serve additive purposes.

The daily reflective sessions provide opportunities for the front line care team to fine tune their daily work together. The weekly team meetings serve a larger purpose as a place where people can make changes together across the entire collaborative care environment. The daily sessions are for day-to-day refinements, whereas the weekly meetings allow for longer term planning and organizational change. Everyone is welcome to attend either meeting. Certain people may want to go to both meetings, while others may choose to go just to one or the other.

Keep showing up

The best way to make collaborative care happen is if the people who are trying to make it happen simply keep showing up every day. At first, if people in the core group advocating for collaborative care are not present on a particular day, other people will almost immediately go right back to their ordinary individual care patterns. Over time, though, if you keep at it, collaborative care will become an expected routine in your care environment. People will miss it if it doesn't happen.

In our research we spoke with a care team member who made this point in a humorous way. He told the story about a day when no one else showed up for rounds. Patients were expecting collaborative care, families were assembled, yet the team wasn't there and no one came except for the one team member, Dan, who was a physical therapy assistant.

Dan was very familiar with collaborative care and often led the rounds process for the team. In our interview with him, he told us that he thought for a while about what to do, then decided to make collaborative rounds anyway, by himself. The irony was not lost on him, of one person making collaborative rounds. But he went through the routines anyway, because he thought it mattered.

He told us that rounds that day was very helpful for many patients and family members, and for himself. Collaborative care had become an essential and expected part of his daily work.

The most important work of the day

In traditional care there are many points where assessments and care decisions are made, most of which happen without the participation of all professions together, and almost always without active participation by patients and families. In this traditional model, rounds often serves as a way of reporting what is already known about a patient's condition, or telling people about a plan that has been already been formulated.

In collaborative care, however, as your team becomes more comfortable working together and actively engaging patients and families, the assessments you make together and the plans you develop together will begin to happen in real time. It will take a while for this to become a new norm, but when it does, your rounds will become much more meaningful and powerful.

One collaborative care team member said, *"In the past, rounds was something that was preparatory for the work of the day, something you had to do before you started your real work. Now, with collaborative rounds, we are realizing that rounds has become our most important work of the day. We do our real work in rounds, and touch up things here and there afterwards."*

This shift, from preparing before rounds and doing your work afterwards, to recognizing that collaborative rounds has become the most important work of the day, is quite significant. People will engage in rounds in a very different way after this shift.

Related to this, or more precisely, during the time before it happens, there will be a tendency of many people to view collaborative rounds as something nice to do for patients, but in fact separate from the real work of patient care. This will be especially true for many physicians. People may want to make their usual "work rounds" first, and collaborative rounds later.

People who have these perspectives are likely to prioritize other things before collaborative rounds if the day heats up. As someone told us, collaborative rounds seems like "fluff," not "core" – nice to do if you have time, but not a true priority.

If collaborative rounds is perceived as "just a nice thing we do for patients and families," but is not felt to be essential for critical parts of care and decision making, it will always feel like a burden to many people. They will have to do their old work and the new work, too. This is likely to show up in conversations as people decide about the right time for collaborative rounds. We often see teams at first envisioning making collaborative rounds later in the day when people "aren't so busy."

These conversations are signs that the care environment is still functioning mostly in traditional ways. We encourage teams to avoid making rounds twice...or three times...or four times. Collaborative rounds becomes truly meaningful and reaches its maximum effectiveness only when it becomes the one central place where assessment and decision making happen.

We advocate strongly that rounds of any kind should happen collaboratively, only once, period. Collaborative rounds should be the only rounds that is done. In later sections we will talk about how preparing for rounds can also be simplified. Nevertheless, it may take some time for people to become comfortable with that. If so, take what you can and work with it. You will eventually get there. But it will be harder to make progress if collaborative rounds begins as a supplemental activity.

Rounds as a scaffolding providing a complete view

In a highly developed collaborative care context, the rounds process itself is an organizing structure that enables the team as a whole, with the patient and family, to inquire together about the patient's condition and other matters of significance.

The rounds process is a scaffolding that allows multiple pieces of information and different observations and perceptions to be assembled into a whole by the combined work of everyone present. The emphasis shifts away from gathering information in preparation for rounds. Instead, everyone brings their small part, and an entire picture is then assembled by everyone together.

Sometimes we use an analogy of decorating a Christmas tree to describe this. Rounds is the bare tree, and each person comes to rounds with an ornament that they hang on the tree, assembling a complete picture of the patient's situation. By these actions an entire picture is assembled that is more complete than any one person could have achieved working individually. The care plan is then built the same way, with everyone participating.

It is important to recognize how profound this shift is regarding the expectations and workflows of each person present. Most health professionals have developed a pattern of data gathering and analysis through years of training and practice that has become familiar and comfortable. It is how they think.

For many people, the pattern of seeing the patient, reviewing the chart, looking at x-rays and laboratory results, and so forth, is often inseparable from how they formulate their understanding of what is happening with the patient and making plans about what to do.

It is not easy at first to switch into a collaborative mode. Transitioning from providing care individually to doing this as a collective team does not happen overnight. It is a learned skill that is part of the work of implementing collaborative care.

In our experience, people will not easily relinquish doing their complete individual preparatory work. Yet gradually they will see that the collaborative picture that emerges is almost always more complete than their very best individual efforts. As they become comfortable trusting that this will happen, they gradually are able to relax into this new and better way of working together. It takes time and experience for this to become evident to people.

Distributed leadership

There is no overstating the need for active engagement of traditional professional leaders as you begin to introduce collaborative rounds. The best way to make collaborative rounds happen is if a respected nurse leader and physician leader arrive on time every day ready to participate in rounds. Showing up that way sends many messages of how important rounds is, and that this new way of working together is a priority. Collaborative rounds is unlikely to succeed without this.

Yet the manner in which leaders engage is important. Role modeling by leaders sets a tone and direction for rounds that will continue long after present leaders are gone, so the way leaders engage is vitally important. We recommend that, very quickly, formal leaders intentionally participate on rounds by being present and engaged, but hand over the role of running rounds to others. Collaborative care requires and thrives on distributed leadership.

Given opportunity and encouragement, many people from across the professions of your team will emerge as advocates and leaders of the rounds process, with special skills and abilities that will energize your rounds. Encouraging many people to take on those leadership roles is wise. They will do an amazing job.

You will notice a different dynamic when a person who is not usually in a formal leadership role runs rounds. This is for at least two reasons, one being the noticeable shift of traditional hierarchy, and the other the professional role cultures of the emerging leaders. For example, a nurse practitioner facilitating rounds will emphasize different things than a physician.

As you make these shifts away from traditional hierarchy, rounds is likely to feel warmer and less formal. New insights will emerge that will surprise you. Invite and welcome this new distributed leadership from within your team.

For many reasons, it may not be easy at first for formal leaders to turn over the leadership of rounds to others. There will often be a tendency of many people on the team to want and expect that kind of traditional direction, and it will be easy for formal leaders to step right up into that directive role. It is what people are used to.

For formal leaders, this requires an interesting balance. Certainly some directive leadership may be beneficial from time to time. But in general, we find that leaders who step back and give others room and time to grow into a distributed leadership model are the most successful. It is helpful for leaders to invite conversations about their ideal role on the team. There is a lot of wisdom among the team if given space for it to come forward.

Direct rounds toward expertise rather than hierarchy

This shift away from the strong assumption in traditional care that the physician will lead and direct the rounds process has interesting aspects. Frequently, in early phases of collaborative care, this expectation of physician leadership carries over to the way that care team members tend to "report" to the physician, and, in more subtle ways, the way patients and family members direct questions to physicians even though other professionals present may have even greater expertise about the answers.

Physicians and other care team members can help to nurture active participation and leadership across the entire care team by inviting people to direct their conversations and questions to the professional team members with greatest expertise in that particular area of concern – for example, respectfully redirecting the conversation to the pharmacist about a medication question, or to the physical therapist about an activity question.

Thoughtful attention by all members of the team to initiate this kind of redirection when questions are asked and to guide the conversation by verbal and non-verbal cues to a different team member's expertise, is powerful. Doing so will quickly lead to a more level hierarchy and a greater sense of level participation for everyone.

Rethinking time

The new work patterns required by collaborative rounds can be quite unsettling in many dimensions for traditional practitioners. At first, doing the work of patient care collaboratively is likely to seem frustratingly slow, painfully unfocused, and irritatingly non-pertinent compared to the comfortable individual workflows that are more familiar and seem much more concise and efficient from the perspective of any single discipline or profession.

In our experience, however, over time the value of collaborative care becomes increasingly apparent for most people. After learning how and becoming proficient at collaborative care, we and most people we have interviewed would never want to go back to their old individual work routines. Collaborative care is much easier and much better. It gives a more complete understanding of what is happening, allows better plans to be made, and assures that things are missed much less often. It is more fun, and takes less time.

But at first, people won't know this. Collaborative care requires learning by experience. It takes experience to see that extra time devoted to collaborative rounds upstream will save time downstream. At first that won't be true. People will have to do their new work and also their old work, which will take extra time.

Gradually, though, that will change and the benefits will be evident. And, as people become more experienced with collaborative care, a shift will begin to happen regarding how people view the time spent on rounds.

With increasing experience, people begin to see that time invested in rounds is usually paid back many times over later in the day. Work that people used to do later can now be done better and more easily during rounds.

People often report finding that they have a significant amount of new time later in the day after spending a moderate amount of extra time to make collaborative rounds together with patients, family members, and other team members. Added to this time savings is less time spent preparing. With savings of time before rounds and after, most people find that the collaborative rounds process is not only better, but more efficient.

Yet health care is busy, even in collaborative care. There is always a time tension, even when collaborative rounds is fully developed. Part of the secret of managing time on rounds is knowing when the collaborative approach needs to give way to individual care later in the day. The collaborative team will learn to sense when the conversation is becoming too focused in any one area, and will learn to respectfully navigate the rounds conversation forward, being sure to acknowledge that a need has not yet been fully met. People can agree to come back later to finish the discussion of that particular point of concern.

With experience, you will be able to sense any developing tension among the team and even among patients and family members when the collaborative rounds process is moving too slowly. The threshold for this tension varies from day to day and situation to situation, but it is real. It is important to monitor this as a team, and to develop ways of respectfully concluding the conversation and moving forward when these moments arise.

You will want to do this intentionally well, taking notice and reflecting about these moments later as a team, because otherwise the tensions of time spent on rounds can lead people to shy away from rounds, or simply to hurry the entire rounds process which usually results in losing its most important benefits.

Practice and reflection make it easier to discern when an investment of time on rounds is necessary, and when individual attention later will work just as well. Certain people are good at recognizing and facilitating these situations, and most teams will soon figure out who among the team members is able to do a particularly good job managing these transitions if invited to do so.

Making thought processes apparent

A significant part of the richness of collaborative rounds is that the intermediate steps of clinical care and decision making are made evident in the rounds conversations. These intermediate steps are the ways in which data and observations are synthesized into insights and actions, and plans are made.

A familiar parallel is the admonition of a math teacher to "show your work." In individual practice the intermediate steps don't usually make it into the medical record and, therefore, are invisible to others in the care environment, including patients and families, who otherwise have only the final outcomes to work with.

In collaborative care these intermediate steps are accomplished in conversations enriched from multiple perspectives. Formative conversations are essential to the work of collaborative care. Because the patient and family members are present and are invited to join in these conversations, they are able to see and participate in this process as it is happening. The same is true for all professional care team members as well.

The benefits of working in these ways are surprisingly deep. First, the understandings and plans that are made are better thought out, because thought processes are apparent and people can see and participate in them. Moreover, the underlying thought processes become part of the care context because people are able to hear the same things over and over, and, they learn.

This accumulated learning makes it easier for everyone – patients, family members, and care team members even in traditional non-clinical roles, such as chaplains or family members – to know what to expect and to recognize problems very early and alert others to any concerns. This is how your care environment moves toward reliability and resilience.

Making thought processes apparent helps to create a web of monitoring that is characteristic of highly evolved collaborative care environments. Both in the care of each individual patient, and in a general sense of knowing what is usually done for every patient, people who participate in collaborative rounds end up being very informed about what is happening, and closely on the same page. Everyone who has participated in rounds knows what is expected for the patient. They are able to recognize departures and concerns, and bring them to the attention of others who can respond, before they become major problems.

Teaching and learning during collaborative rounds

The essence of collaborative care is teaching and learning. At times, every person in the collaborative environment will be a teacher, and a learner. And, the entire care environment is constantly learning. The environment teaches, too, as new people come and socialize by conversations and interactions into “how things are done around here.” Participating in collaborative care is an ongoing learning experience of the highest order.

In an environment centered on teaching and learning, it should be easy for people to take time to intentionally teach. There are so many interested people present at collaborative rounds, and so much wisdom and experience to share.

In practice, though, it may take a while for comfort with formal teaching and learning to become a part of your collaborative care routines. It is our experience that people may be concerned at first that others in other professions may not be interested in what would be taught, or may not want to take the time required. And, professional team members may not realize that patients and families are usually very interested and capable of learning about their care from a professional perspective.

Teaching and learning raises the environment for everyone. Although you may have to intentionally step forward and try it, when you do, we believe you will be delighted and possibly surprised by how receptive people are, and how much they appreciate the time that others are willing to invest.

The beauty of a collaborative care environment is that any teaching is absorbed and has a place where it can be remembered and used again. Things once learned by the collaborative team are not forgotten. You will see teaching come back to you very quickly in grateful people and improved care.

Emergence

A hallmark of collaborative care is the emergence of new ideas and insights on rounds and during team meetings. The emergence of new ideas and insights as the care team interacts and converses is part of the "generativity" of collaborative care. This property of emergence is very important for resilience.

In the same way that assessment occurs collaboratively in real time, the development of a care plan occurs in real time as well. Ideas for care arise in conversations and are tested and improved as they are developed and agreed upon.

The benefits of collaborative rounds are not simply because everyone who is present knows the care plan. The picture of what is happening, and the plans that are made, are richer, more insightful, and more effective when they are made collaboratively, especially when patients and families are included, than if they are made only by a part of the care team in isolation.

In our research and practice, it is notable that new ideas emerge in the course of rounds conversations that were not in the mind of any one person when the rounds conversation began. One person's thought or observation triggers another person's idea, and from this interplay between people, new ideas emerge that weren't there before the conversation started.

Distributing power (leveling)

Power is a topic that deserves careful thought regarding collaborative rounds and collaborative care in general. There are so many ways that power is woven throughout the interactions, expectations, hopes, and fears of everyone involved in collaborative care processes.

In traditional health care, asymmetries of power are present and expected, in particular around the physician role and the presumed expertise of health care professionals in relation to patients and families. There are multi-generational stories about power and its evolution, such as the emergence of nursing as a profession in response to power inequalities, and connections with broader societal concerns and discourses such as gender.

The purpose of this section is not to enter deeply into these considerations; however, it is important to keep in mind that the experiences of power in health care have deep parallels in society as a whole, and at any moment and within any team there will be multiple histories, multiple personal stories, many emotions, and the likelihood of notably divergent perspectives, expectations, and beliefs about power.

After many years of work with collaborative care, we now recognize that power is a paradox. No single understanding of power is sufficient, and the experiences of power are complex. However, it is clear there is a trajectory toward a different kind of power in collaborative care.

Collaborative care benefits from certain aspects of power, such as specialized knowledge in which trust may be placed and counted on, yet it expresses power in ways that do not carry as many of the frequent harmful effects.

In collaborative care the differences between roles are able to be held in ways that change the attributes of power having to do with "authority over" and "control of" people. Care becomes more inviting and participatory. To describe this shift we have chosen to use the word, "leveling."

In a leveling way, power in collaborative care is something co-created by people who are working together as "just people." At a practical level these shifts take place through simple human actions, such as sitting with a patient rather than standing, listening with attention, inviting contributions, devoting time, showing interest, and encouraging emerging power as it develops throughout the assembled group.

Contributions become richer, interactions become more generative, and the focus and purpose of the work becomes more human. Another dimension of the power paradox is that, even as role hierarchy levels, role differences become even more valuable.

For professionals in roles that could expect hierarchical authority in traditional health care, such as physicians, this leveling of hierarchy requires some changes in thinking. It soon becomes apparent for many people that working in a collaborative way leads to more authentic valuing by others.

Whatever power might be lost through leveling of hierarchy is replaced by authentic respect and appreciation created in a new way. The satisfactions of role hierarchy are replaced in collaborative care by a different and remarkably more rewarding bond of mutual respect and shared achievement between members of the care team, patients, and family members.

The shift toward level hierarchy has another benefit, often unexpected, of an increased human focus over technical aspects of care. As people begin to interact as "just people" rather than from hierarchical professional roles, the environment takes on a notably more human-centered character.

Leveling of hierarchy makes it possible for the care team to accomplish technical and scientific aspects of care in exceptional ways. They have never been done as well.

Yet, in highly evolved collaborative care, the technical and scientific aspects of care are seen from a new perspective as part of a greater whole, and are no longer viewed as the only essential goal or primary purpose.

What about people who don't like working this way?

Existing power dynamics in health care are strong, and in our experience there will be uncomfortable moments for the newly forming collaborative team regarding power. For example, it is likely that your team will include physicians and nursing leaders who are excited about collaborative care, and others who view the world from a more traditional professional perspective that expects the physician or executive to direct, and others to follow.

When a collaborative care team interacts with traditional practitioners and managers, for example when a team is engaged in a collaborative conversation with a patient and family, and a physician who has not been part of providing care this way comes to see the patient at the same time, we have observed that people will not know at first how to manage the different worlds that are coexisting. An awkwardness may linger afterward, as people struggle to sort out the unspoken conflicts of actions and priorities they have just experienced.

As collaborative care is getting started, it is not unusual for traditional managers to restrict people from participating in rounds because of a perceived need for meeting traditional productivity goals. This can be stressful for people who see the benefits of collaborative care and feel allegiances to the collaborative team, but who also work in traditional reporting relationships.

Situations like this are learning opportunities for the collaborative team if people are courageous and confident enough to talk about what is happening, and especially if they can do so with an open heart and a receptive understanding. Collaborative care is not the same as traditional practice, and the differences are strikingly apparent in circumstances like this.

The most helpful insights we have observed when discussing situations like this come from remembering that almost everyone in health care is trying to do the best they can to take care of patients in ways that make sense to them. The doctor or manager who directs rather than collaborates is working from an understanding that directing is what they are supposed to do. The same is true of health care professionals who have achieved mastery in their traditional roles and don't see a need to change.

The vulnerabilities of collaborative care are evident in interactions such as these. Power asymmetries may be painfully apparent when understandings differ. In environments of traditional power, collaborative care can be stopped by the dissenting voice of a physician, or the opposition of formal or informal nursing leaders and others, including administrators, if they choose to act to oppose the collaborative care process.

When these kinds of conflicts happen, our advice is just to regroup as a care team, seek out people who are interested in this work, and find ways to keep going. It may take a while to regain forward progress, but almost always, circumstances change and you can make progress again.

Early on, we tried to convert people to collaborative care. Later we found it was more effective to "work with the willing" rather than convert the opposed. Much of the work we have done since then has been accomplished from this wiser perspective.

Seek out the viewpoints of others, listen carefully, and invite them to experience what you are doing. Do so out of strength, with respect for the people involved. Model in your actions that differences are welcome here. Over time, as you do, collaborative ways of working will become stronger and stronger.

What to expect

In our experience, at first collaborative rounds will seem to take forever. People are likely to be interested, but also will worry about getting all their own work done. There will be a time tension at first for many people.

As your team continues to work together, collaborative care will start to become more comfortable. People will begin to see that devoting time on rounds and in meetings saves time later in the day. A good thing will be how much your patients and family members appreciate what you are doing. That will be very evident very soon, and will probably be enough for people to keep trying.

Gradually, a change will happen in your care environment. People will begin to experience that working collaboratively is more rewarding than the ways your team used to work. You will learn things about other professions you didn't realize you didn't know. You will form deeper relationships with patients and family members than you ever experienced before.

Your work will become more meaningful, more like what you hoped a health care profession would be. And your outcomes and patient satisfaction will skyrocket in ways you always hoped could be possible. The outcome changes and satisfaction shifts will startle you. You will say, "We didn't know this was possible."

In time, most people will appreciate many things about collaborative care. They will notice they have a better understanding of what is happening with the patients, and they know what is planned. They won't have to call each other as much during the day. Work will become easier and more rewarding.

There will be a growing sense of professionalism, and a growing appreciation for being recognized for each person's contributions. There will also be a new sense of compassion. Family members will stop being so worried. There will be almost no "problem families."

Patients will relax more, and will be less sick. They will participate more in their own care, with surprising confidence. If things go wrong, people will catch things sooner and the team will be able to get things back on track sooner. All of these things will start to be evident to people. You can expect the medical part of your work to get smaller, and the human part of your work to have new meaning. You can expect to form new friendships with your professional colleagues, and to forge lifelong friendships with your patients. You can expect to go home renewed most days instead of often feeling depleted and exhausted.

All of this will take about eighteen months if you follow the advice in this field guide. Yes, all of this will really happen. But...

Always challenges

These changes will almost certainly occur, but there will be plenty of challenges along the way. You should not expect that collaborative care will be easy to achieve. Some people will like working in these new ways, and others won't. It will be emotionally difficult. Things will move forward, then slide back. Frustrating!

Competing concerns will arise that will take time and attention away from your work together. New people will join your team who will not be familiar with your work. Leaders will change, bringing their own ideas.

To be perfectly honest, it takes a lot of courage to implement collaborative care. Health care is a very complex landscape, with multiple forces contending for a future that is not yet written, in the context of a past that is dying but not yet dead.

Many people and most organizations in health care find their purposes in the roles and patterns they have worked hard to acquire and have become accustomed to. As you implement collaborative care, you will inevitably touch hearts and minds both for better and for worse, and unintentionally trample on identities.

When these things happen, and they will, remember that almost always the best way to meet these challenges is by going forward together. Invite people to participate. Give people the choice of being present when they can. Be resilient, patient, and persistent. Be willing to listen, reflect, reevaluate, and change.

You will need to patiently invite and welcome people into your work and the progress you have made, time and time again.

Keep trying.

Down the road, you will be very glad you did things this way. Your social field will reflect the care and devotion that you commit to it in these early stages. The spirit and nature that you show in every action and decision you make, especially in adversity, is being woven into the new culture you are creating.

Laughter as a marker of collaborative care

Collective attention to "holding shared space together" is very important for the rounds process to be effective at every level, including an emotional level. This means that everyone's attention is focused on having a shared, respectful conversation.

As the team begins to shift into a mode of meaningful collective work together, there are noticeable changes in the interactions. One consistent finding we see is that laughter starts happening on rounds as collaborative care develops. Laughter is an unmistakable marker that a care team is becoming comfortable working with each other and with patients and families.

At first it might seem unusual, even inappropriate, for care teams to laugh with each other and with patients and families during rounds. After all, this is often happening in an intensive care unit. However, with collaborative care, it is quite common. When we asked one team about their laughter, people said, "It is comfortable laughter, not nervous laughter. We just really like working this way together."

Comfortable laughter on rounds indicates that people are working at a level of rich human connections. In our experience, laughter happens frequently in collaborative care. The emergence of natural, respectful attentiveness and responsiveness of the entire team together, including laughter, is an important marker of the development of your collaborative care environment. Take note of the laughter. You will see it very early in your work.

Summary of things your team can do to develop collaborative rounds

A consistent pattern for daily collaborative care can be intentionally developed by a particular care team in their own ways. This pattern for working together can become consistent and predictable, allowing people to know what to expect in most situations, how to respond, and how to coordinate with one another. Having a pattern makes routine care easier, and enables the team to devote special care and attention to what is unique about each patient and family.

- Your team can intentionally develop a collaborative pattern for working together that your team can become very familiar with and that you know will happen consistently every day.

- You can strive to align your schedules so that everyone is able to be together for rounds, and if someone can't be there, then someone else can represent that role in a planned way.

- You can intentionally make care decisions when your team is all together and patients and families are present.
- You can establish a team norm that people are not expected as individuals to know everything before rounds – instead you can encourage people to each bring their part and then your rounds process assembles the parts into a complete picture.
- You can use a whiteboard in the patient's room to record your work together. As you develop your plan, write it down where it can be seen and review it before you leave the room.
- You can develop a safety checklist to use as part of your rounds process with every patient. The checklist is a prompt for important things you want to be sure you do every time.
- You can reflect with your team about learning to work together; for example, your team may find it is difficult at first to keep attention focused on team conversations, and then it becomes a lot easier.
- You can intentionally ask patients, family members, and yourselves as a routine part of your collaborative care process if anything that happened was unexpected, or if you could do things differently or better.
- You can reflect with your team about whether you have learned about others across professional roles as you have developed a collaborative structure for your work together.
- You can reflect with your team about whether new collaborative care routines allow your team to do the ordinary things effortlessly together, with time and energy left over for devoting attention to what is special about each patient.

Active Engagement of Patients and Families

A significant difference between traditional practice and collaborative care is active engagement of patients and families in all aspects of care and decision making. In order to accomplish this, patients and families must function as engaged and essential members of the care team, not separate from it.

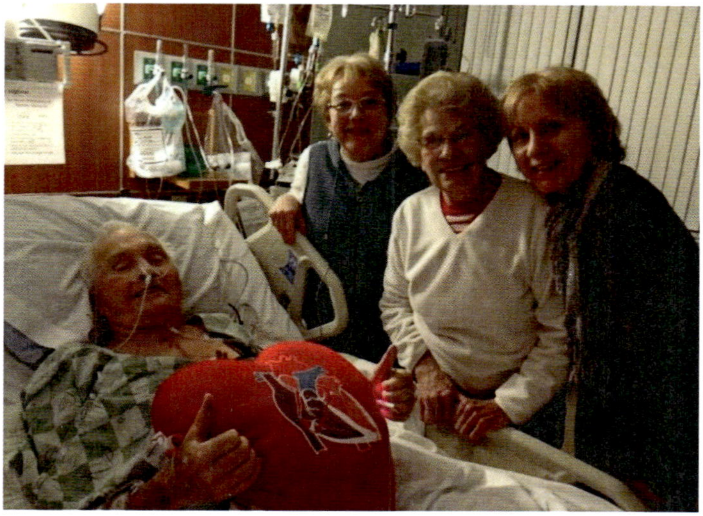

Photo: Clarence and his family

Inviting and welcoming patients and families by other members of the care team can create these bonds of connection in a short period of time, opening the team to active engagement by patients and family members.

Relational bridges can be intentionally established that transcend expectations and past experiences of professional distance and asymmetries of specialized medical knowledge. The actions that accomplish this are, on the one hand, very simple, and yet on the other hand, remarkably powerful in their symbolic nature and practical effect.

The process of opening the team to active engagement by patients and families starts before rounds begins, as people start to congregate for rounds. We advocate thoughtfully and intentionally not having conversations about the patient outside the door of the room, in hallways, or in conference areas where patients and families cannot participate.

Once together with the patient, words and actions that invite and welcome patients and families into care continue with invitations, and how people stand or sit, and position themselves.

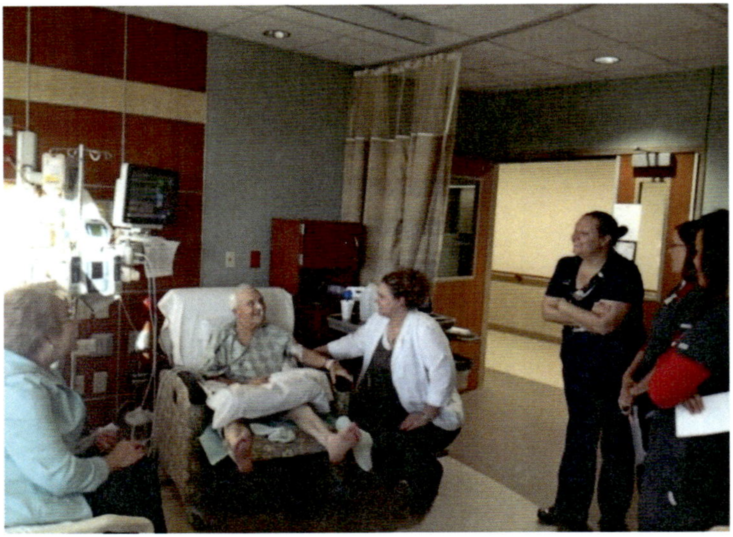

Photo: Inviting active engagement of patients and families

Nonverbal actions of smiles, making eye contact, respectful touching, the directions in which people turn, gestures and facial expressions, the kind of language used, and the cadence and pacing of conversations are all very important.

Patients and families are watching the actions of the care team closely. Everything your team does is a signal to patients and family members about what is about to happen next. Words and actions can be chosen that invite active engagement and indicate inclusion and welcoming of patients and families into the inner workings of care.

Doing this requires careful, thoughtful attention, because traditional patterns of interaction on rounds, and the specialized language often used in health care, are deeply ingrained from years of training and experience.

You can hear this in the usual patterns and words used, such as talking among the team about patients in the third person saying "she" or "he" in a mode of reporting, rather than speaking directly with the patient saying "you." This can also be recognized as a team physically turns inward toward each other away from the patient and family, talking among themselves about the patient even though the patient is right there and could participate.

It can be hard at first for clinical teams to change these patterns, or even to be aware of them, because of how deeply these traditional ways of working are used throughout the everyday interactions and routines of most people in health care.

When intentional efforts are made to change these patterns, the least experienced members of the care team, such as students, are often able to adopt the new patterns most easily, whereas experienced team members usually find it harder, often lapsing back into traditional "reporting" mode without realizing it.

The reason we are devoting so much attention to these distinctions is because the way that patients and families respond to care interactions is significantly influenced by these patterns. Yet, traditional patterns are so familiar that most care teams do not normally stop to think about them and their effects. Relatively minor changes in these patterns can produce remarkable benefits.

The initial stress of engaging patients and families

As researchers, we often see that, as care teams begin collaborative care, there may be a reluctance to emphasize participation of patients and families.

If we ask why a team is reluctant to actively include patients and families at these early formative stages, there is often an uncomfortable response. People tell us they understand that engagement of patients and families is their long term goal, but trying to do that "right now" is just too hard. Professional care team members often say that the stress of having conversations among themselves across professions is high enough already.

People also worry about how much time it will take to involve patients and families. In traditional care this would be true, because there is so much "pent up" anxiety. In our experience, collaborative care takes this anxiety away quickly, and the time it takes to do this becomes minor quickly as everyone becomes comfortable. But a care team won't know this as they first begin.

Another feeling that teams express is embarrassment. Professional care team members say they would be uncomfortable and embarrassed if patients and families actually knew how imperfect and disconnected things really are.

Our observations have shown that there is a tendency in traditional health care practice of wanting to have everything figured out, and everyone on the same page, before interacting with the patient or family members. It is sometimes said, "We have to be aligned and certain so we do not shake their confidence."

This sense of wanting to have everything in order before including patients and families is especially evident in the moments before the team enters a patient's room for rounds. This takes many forms in traditional health care practice, from a quick exchange between colleagues before rounds, to an extensive conversation outside the door before entering the room, to detailed care planning in meetings among multiple specialties and professions. Teams traditionally meet and talk together outside the room to prepare before being with patients and families.

Unspoken in these meetings is a host of expectations in traditional health care practice related to assumptions about expertise of health care professionals, and an assumption that trust arises from this expertise. Practitioners have been taught that trust and optimum practitioner-patient relationships depend on knowing and projecting confidence about what is best.

Inviting and welcoming into comfortable authenticity

Everyone knows the experience of cleaning the floor, dusting the furniture, and polishing the mirror in the bathroom before opening our homes to others. People live in comfortable ways that we imagine would be embarrassing if others could see us and judge us as we really are.

The tendency of wanting to be carefully prepared before meeting with patients and family members is a natural human tendency. But it unintentionally holds teams and patients apart.

Collaborative care is based upon comfortable authenticity. At its best, collaborative care encourages teams to build care environments they are comfortable sharing with patients and families on a moment's notice without advance preparation.

Collaborative care invites us to be simply who we are as people, welcoming each other into all the difficult realities and uncertainties of health care. Collaborative care is like having best friends stop by unexpectedly and welcoming them with arms wide open, without a thought about anything except the friendship. It is imperfect, sometimes a mess, and that is just fine.

What is made possible by "welcoming into authenticity"? In such a context, people are free to respond unburdened by unnecessary and unrealistic expectations. New ideas and insights are more able to emerge from such interactions.

Over time, as the capability for trusting one another grows among people, an even greater comfort arises. The environment takes on a more personal character and is increasingly filled with new meaning and aliveness. Collaborative care weaves the inevitable disorder of health care into a "wonderfully imperfect" fabric of human authenticity, trust, and potential.

Taking time

We advocate changing patterns of interaction on rounds so that patients and families are able to actively engage and truly be part of the care team. If we are asked to point to one central goal of the new patterns of interaction we are advocating, that goal would be "taking time."

The most important thing a team can do to actively engage patients and families in care is to take time – time to welcome, time to listen, and time to authentically include patients and families in care. It seems like this should be simple, yet at first it may seem impossibly hard to take the time to do these things well.

The patterns we advocate for rounds, for example the patterns of beginning with introductions around the circle, and of going around the circle again to be sure that everyone present has an opportunity to contribute, are rhythms that "make time."

The patterns and rhythms of collaborative care presented in this and other sections are relational technologies. Utilizing the rounds guide on pages 118 and 119 will open your team to active engagement by patients and families through the patterns and rhythms that the use of the guide will establish in your rounds.

It may be tempting to skip ahead of the rhythms as you are trying out these new patterns. They will seem too slow at first. But if you do skip ahead past the rhythms, you will compress the time you are making and inadvertently lose the benefits that the rhythms will produce. If, though, you hold onto the new patterns, you will soon discover that taking time actually makes time. This may seem paradoxical at first, but it is true. As your care team finds ways and takes time to open itself to active engagement by patients and families, the nature of every interaction changes.

Conversations become more peaceful, tensions lessen, mutual respect grows, and the experiences of care become more efficient and more meaningful. Rounds may take a little longer, but the rest of the day and each subsequent day will be shorter, easier, and better.

Worried about his dog

There is a story from a collaborative care team that helps bring to life what happens as patients and family are actively included in care. The story concerns a patient who was not doing well after heart surgery. He was a farmer who lived alone in the woods. His nearest neighbor lived several miles away. His operation had gone very well and everything measureable about his recovery was coming along fine. His laboratory values and chest x-ray were normal, his vital signs were normal. But he was not eating well, and was not walking. He was growing weaker and beginning to have difficulty coughing and clearing his lungs. Everyone on the care team could see his deterioration and worried about him. No one knew what should be done differently.

One morning during collaborative rounds someone noted on the goal board that the patient had a dog. When the dog was mentioned the patient's eyes lighted up for a brief moment, then tears came to his eyes. The social worker comforted him and the team listened attentively as she asked him about his dog. He loved his dog. His dog was his family. When he came into the hospital he had left his dog with his neighbor, but he had not been able to talk with his neighbor since his surgery. He was literally worried sick about his dog. His most important goal was making sure his dog was OK. He didn't know how to do that. His worry occupied his thoughts. The team was able to send the sheriff to check on his neighbor. His dog was fine. The next day the patient was much better, and several days later he was able to go home.

Time after time during our research and practice, we have heard stories like this, of things that came to light involving or beyond the medical care that made all the difference because of active engagement of patients and families. This patient wanted to go to his sister's wedding. This patient wanted to see her son play in a special football game. This father knew his daughter needed a special blanket. This family knew their sister was having a stroke because her unusual symptoms were just like what their brother had. This son knew that his father was having a life-threatening reaction that wasn't listed as an allergy. This wife knew that her husband would never take a particular medicine because his father had died after taking it. This mother knew that if the emergency room doctor would only call the urologist who had operated on her daughter, they would be able to send her home.

In each of these stories, taking time and listening made all the difference. In many, the listening happened early and well during exemplary collaborative care. In others, the listening finally happened after a lot of unnecessary anxiety and stress during care in an older model. In every case, care improved a lot after everyone was engaged, listening, talking, and deciding together.

"Prepared but Incomplete"

We advocate thoughtfully minimizing the amount of preparation that is done before rounds. The goal is to do just enough preparing to be sure that important facts are brought to rounds, but to intentionally keep assessment "incomplete" and not make any plans until patients, family members, and the rest of the care team can be present to actively assess and plan together.

There is an expectation in traditional health care that everyone coming to rounds must be thoroughly prepared ahead of time. This is part of the intense individual accountability that is woven throughout traditional health care practice and education.

The result of this traditional expectation is that patients are awakened very early in the morning by each individual participant in their care. In teaching institutions the medical student sees the patient very early, the first year resident comes shortly after, then the senior resident, then the fellow, and so on. The same is true for each of the other health professions team members.

In addition to pre-rounds, important planning conversations often occur separate from the patient and family in a conference room, at a counter or table in the intensive care unit, or outside the patient's room. Plans made by a physician or a resident team may be passed along to other care team members primarily by orders entered into the patient record. Often the patient is unaware of these plans or is informed of them as they unfold.

In our research and practice, gradually at first and then with increasing clarity, we recognized that it is better to wait until everyone can be present, including patients and family members, before trying to synthesize a picture of what is happening, and before making care plans.

You might be thinking, as we did, that it should be helpful to have a pre-rounds team meeting or a morning huddle before starting the day. Aren't those supposed to be best practices? Isn't it good for the team to meet and talk?

Gradually we began to recognize that whenever part of a team meets and talks together, understandings are being formed. The understandings created by these conversations depend on who is present and talking together. If patients, families, and other professions are not present and involved in these conversations, the understandings that are developed will not fully reflect these missing insights, contributions, needs, and beliefs.

We have seen in our research that pre-work and having separate conversations before rounds have the unintended result of excluding important professional viewpoints and limiting engagement of patients and families in assessment and planning.

This may seem puzzling at first to care team members who are used to touching base before rounds, informing one another of things that have happened, and checking about this or that. To explore this, try waiting until your team is all together with patients and families before having care conversations, then see if you can tell a difference.

In our experience, it is surprising how much the "pre-conversations" shape interactions and decision making in ways that weren't apparent. By waiting until everyone is together, details and insights emerge that wouldn't have been thought of without everyone there, including the patient and family. You might be surprised how important these are. We certainly were.

This is especially true regarding patient and family contributions. We began to recognize that a care team by itself cannot completely know the concerns and hopes of patients and families. We thought we were representing the concerns and goals of our patients and families well in our care meetings without them. Over time, we began to see that something better was possible. With increasing experience, we began to recognize the importance of active participation by patients and family members in every team conversation and care decision.

These differences are not minor. It is startling to realize how much the active participation of patients and families adds to care, and how often it changes the understandings that are reached and the decisions and the actions that are taken.

It is hard to recognize this at first for most teams. In traditional culture it may seem proper to make assessments and decisions on behalf of patients, especially when a care team perceives that a patient is hard to deal with, or if there is a "problem" patient or family member. It is hard at first to realize how much the perceptions of the care team are formed and maintained by these separate conversations, and how different they often are when patients and families are present.

More significantly, we now see that by meeting and talking among ourselves separately from our patients we were unintentionally creating and perpetuating divisions of knowledge and power between ourselves and our patients. We had no idea we were doing that.

Without realizing it, the actions of having "the conversation before the conversation," unintentionally build distance. With good intentions, assumptions are being made about what patients and families want. Yet the absence of patient and family voices in these conversations means that whatever is being decided in these conversations does not fully include them.

The insights that are reached and the decisions that are made are notably better when care is truly collaborative and unfolds in real time. In our research and practice we have seen how different the conversations on rounds become when all voices are included in every activity.

Just people together – lessening professional distance

In our experience, collaborative care often begins with a degree of tension about engaging patients and families. Farther down the road toward collaborative care, when sensitivities change and awareness is greater, it is possible for teams to recognize how much was missing and inaccessible when they prepared for rounds without participation of the patient and family.

Remember that we're talking about a journey toward collaborative care. At the beginning of the journey, care teams and the patients and families they care for are surrounded by present ways of understanding care and the expectations of those ways.

For patients and families, traditional understandings carry many expectations. There is often a reluctance of patients and families to impose upon the time of the care team. There is a hesitancy to ask questions or to be fully forthcoming about concerns, and a reluctance to be transparent as patients and families may choose or want a different course of action than the one advised but hesitate to say anything.

These traditional expectations are held by the care team as well. There is a reluctance to express not knowing. There is a desire to prepare ahead of time and to present a confident and certain demeanor. There is a belief in the value of maintaining objective distance and keeping professional involvement separate from any real personal relationship.

Any intent of actively engaging patients and families in care begins from this starting place. Over time, with deeper insight, a new kind of inviting and welcoming without the burden of embarrassment makes possible different kinds of conversations among care teams, patients and family members in which everything has changed.

In place of worries about what the patient might think comes a new comfort. In place of unspoken mistrust comes a new acceptance and forgiveness. The power of active engagement with patients and families, and its freshness, is startling.

One patient said, “You treated us like ordinary people, and that made all the difference.”

Treating people as well, not sick

One of the most interesting shifts we have observed regarding collaborative care is the emergence and growth of an orientation away from sickness care toward a different approach to care that emphasizes strengths and capabilities.

Although the medical details of the care of each patient are addressed very carefully, a highly developed collaborative care environment allows these details to be accomplished much more effectively than in traditional care, in ways that create time and space for additional areas of attention.

Also, active engagement of patients and families is a naturally stronger role than in traditional care. Taken together these changes have the effect of shifting attention from what is missing or wrong, to what is right.

As teams first begin to work collaboratively these changes are often surprising. Patients become less sick.

A story is helpful here. Several years after implementing collaborative care on a cardiac surgery unit, the care team gave a presentation at another hospital about their work and their improved outcomes.

After the team described actively engaging patients and families on daily collaborative rounds, a physician in the audience asked, "Well, that may be fine for the well patients, but what about the sick ones?" The team members looked at one another and thoughtfully replied, "These are the same patients we have always cared for. They are the same patients you care for, too. They just aren't sick in the same way anymore." This answer did not make sense to the physician, who had never experienced care like this.

Everything changes

The traditional education process of becoming a health professional involves learning to understand the condition of a patient from a highly nuanced framework of applied medical science and nursing practice with deep traditions.

For physicians, these traditions honor the art of medicine which is held alongside the science of medicine as equally important and taking years to master. Over time, the art of medicine has come to be viewed as something nice but less essential than the science – for example taking a careful history so that an accurate diagnosis can be made.

Similarly in the profession of nursing, the human actions of touching and bathing and bandaging and feeding and providing fresh bedding have gradually been given over to others, providing more time for professional responsibilities of assessment, nursing diagnosis, coordination of care, communicating and documenting.

The unintended consequence of this focus on medical science and professional nursing practice is a longing by patients and professionals alike for a reawakening of awareness that health care is actually about human connections.

What becomes central in collaborative care is care itself, care in its most basic and human form. It is very simple, really. As human beings we recognize care by remembering our most central relationships. Care is devotion. Care is listening and watching with full attention. Care is protecting. Care is stepping back, and letting go. Care is celebrating.

In highly evolved collaborative care, the human interactions of care are reciprocal rather than flowing only in one direction. Care and expertise flow freely where they are needed, among and throughout everyone present. This can happen only when a true leveling has occurred.

Rather than an exhausting one-way flow of giving, the human-centered give and take of collaborative care is often filled with every human emotion, including joy and laughter.

Participating in this kind of exchange is healing and restorative for everyone.

A circle of mutual care and respect

What patients remember after care of any kind, traditional or collaborative, is moments of human connection. In collaborative care, conversations become possible across professions that involve patients and families. The needs, hopes and fears of patients are able to be heard clearly and strongly. Similarly, the opportunity for practitioners to interact in new ways with patients and families is restorative for care givers.

Patients and families receive care, but they also provide care for their providers, with a richness of new connections and new meaning that changes what it is like to be a nurse or a doctor.

Similarly, patients and families are able to experience a different kind of care that touches them at a level of meaning not available in most traditional experiences. At first, these shifts seemed exceptional to us, but we now realize that they are simply what happens when hierarchies become level, and patients and families are able to actively engage in co-creating care.

No longer is expertise in health care simply about medical or professional knowledge. Instead, a different kind of expertise arises that is much more mutual. It exists across the entire team, including the patient and family members, and is based on awareness of the needs, hopes, and expectations of everyone involved. With this growing insight comes surprising tolerance, forgiveness, interest, and mutual support. One patient family member that we interviewed described this as a “crossing over.” She made a gesture with her hands, rolling them over and opening her fingers to show reciprocity. She meant that the needs of the patient became the needs of the care team, and the needs of the care team became the needs of the patient and family.

In collaborative care there is a merging of interests and abilities between the care team and the patient and the family. The purpose of care becomes helping people live intact and meaningful lives. The patient and family help the care team as much as the care team helps the patient and family. Care becomes reciprocal, co-created between people working together.

A purpose of meaning in a context of human connections

The patient centered care movement is an attempt to acknowledge the asymmetries of power and information in traditional health care practice and to give greater control and greater attention to the participation and informed decision making of the patient, often with recognition of the importance of families.

There is a desire to remember and honor the relationship between patient and practitioner, and an intention of most teams of becoming even more patient-centered. Even so, underlying models often remain strongly oriented toward scientific and technical care, often with a goal of "educating" patients so they can make more knowledgeable scientific and technical decisions. Implied often is a notably unidirectional give and take relationship between care providers and care consumers, with the flow of giving directed toward the patient as "delivery" of care by "providers" to "consumers."

Taken to an extreme, this model is depleting. As more and more is asked of nurses, doctors, social workers, and others providing care in this model, with greater and greater expectations and workload, it is no wonder that people feel exhausted and empty at the end of the day rather than restored and renewed.

Health care should be one of the most fulfilling and rewarding of human experiences. Yet, often in present care, and even in well intended alternatives, it ends up being just the opposite. From the perspective of patients, very often these innovations still feel alienating. Something is still missing. And for the practitioner there can be a sense of self-sacrifice about patient-centeredness – that the needs and wellbeing of the patient must come before all other concerns. At limits, this self-sacrifice can be depleting and exhausting.

Well down the road toward collaborative care, a deeper and different kind of engagement between health professionals, patients, and families emerges that supports a surprisingly different understanding and experience of patient centered care.

Collaborative care is not a delivery model. Collaborative care is meaning-centered, and is co-created among people who are working together to care for each other. Care itself becomes the focus, not simply science as the focus. We describe this as, "a purpose of meaning, in a context of human connections."

When this kind of care is the goal, then a health care system that is sustainable and renewable becomes possible to imagine. As we give, we also receive. Collaborative care restores care givers as much as the people they care for. Care from this perspective turns out to be an infinitely renewable resource.

Summary of things your team can do to actively engage patients and families

Teams can intentionally open the care environment to the interests, preferences, and contributions of patients and family members. Structures and routines can be developed that actively engage patients and families in care, such as encouraging visiting at any time, and inviting and welcoming participation of patients and family members in collaborative rounds.

- You can create policies that encourage family members to be present at any time, and invite and welcome patients and families to participate in care and decision making.

- You can invite and welcome patients and family members to participate as members of your team on daily rounds, and encourage them to join the circle and contribute.

- You can intentionally avoid trying to "get your house in order" before seeing and talking with patients and families – do things in real time with everyone involved from the beginning.

- During rounds, you can make it a first priority to ask about the lives and interests of the patient and family. Write those down on the whiteboard as part of your record.

- Try to make no assumptions about what patients and families want or need until you ask them – and be intentional about asking as part of the routines you are developing.

- You can be aware of how you stand, and encourage ordinary language so that your actions and your words help patients and families feel included in what you are doing together.

- You can be intentional about not telling people what to do, or even what they should do – instead ask, listen, and decide together what is best and what to do.

- You can talk openly with patients and families about everything that is happening – if there are errors or mistakes or uncertainties, you can make your concerns transparent.

- You can take note of how your understanding of your work grows as you involve patients and families – discuss the surprising changes because of it.

- You can form a patient/family advisory council and encourage members from this council to attend your system meetings and work as partners to improve care.

PART FIVE

DEEPENING

- Action-Reflection Learning Systems
    - Down and In Data
    - GLITCH Process
- The Benefits of Team Learning
- Evolution of the Collaborative Care Environment
- Achieving Reliability and Resilience

Action-Reflection Learning Systems

Very often we find that people are interested in implementing collaborative rounds, but have not fully thought about how the benefit of rounds depends on the ability of the care team to learn together, and to apply what they have learned in reliable and resilient ways. Collaborative rounds is important. However, achieving exceptional collaborative care depends on creating a care environment that supports team-level learning. Collaborative rounds is a part of that, but maybe a third at most.

The main lesson of our work is that the focus of implementation efforts should be on the care environment as a whole, not just on rounds. The goal should be to create an environment that is ideally optimized for team-level learning and system improvement. If you approach collaborative care in this broader way, you will accomplish more and are more likely to be successful. Reliability and resilience require team-level learning that enriches the abilities carried and applied in your social field.

In this section our emphasis is on collaborative learning in social fields, and structural ways that the capacities for team-level learning can be supported and enhanced. To understand how collaborative care deepens and develops toward reliability and resilience, it is useful to consider a care team together with its social field as comprising an "action-reflection learning system."

Collaborative care emerges best in a certain kind of curiosity-filled, psychologically safe environment where learning can thrive. In a well-developed social field the knowledge that enables exceptional performance grows and is applied by the care team as a whole. This shift of focus from the individual to the collective as the "unit of analysis" is essential for understanding how reliability and resilience emerge through team learning.

As a first step, consistency of interactions is foundational for team learning. Without consistency of interactions, today's team is not tomorrow's team. Whatever might be learned from today's interactions cannot be applied tomorrow unless there is some kind of continuity. This is a foundational principle.

A brief story helps to illustrate this. Consider an intensive care unit that was established by a group of people who have a long history of working together extremely well. Everyone in this particular care unit knows its history, can recall major events that have happened through the years, and knows the personalities and strengths of one another.

Now, imagine that a massive staff turnover happens, perhaps people retire, or a staffing reduction happens. The unit is now staffed by equally qualified practitioners, but these people have no history together and many have been brought in for brief assignments. People don't even know where to find supplies. By the time they do learn, they are rotated off the unit to other floors.

What would it be like to work in this unit before and after the staff turnover? In the first case, the environment would be rich with tacit knowledge. In the second case, the tacit knowledge would be very limited. No matter how much a team might try to work well together, in the second case its performance would be notably limited until tacit knowledge was rebuilt and useful again.

The point of this example is to direct attention to the team level, to the attributes of teams and care environments that enable team-level learning, and to the importance of team-level learning for building tacit knowledge. The capabilities of exceptional collaborative care develop over time as the care team advances to ever higher levels of collective performance through ongoing team-level learning that produces rich "know-how" of the team.

How team learning happens

As a place to begin our thinking, let's consider how an individual learns and becomes really good at something. In a minute, we'll take this from an individual level to the entire team.

Most people have something they enjoy and want to learn how to do well. For example, a person might enjoy woodworking. Many skills are needed to be an expert woodworker. There are basic skills that can be learned from a book, and there are additional, more complex skills that require time and experience to learn.

Let's watch a person learning how to do complex woodworking. The person already has basic skills. To take those skills to the next level, the woodworker needs to learn.

We are in the woodworking shop. The woodworker has carefully prepared, and is ready to make something that requires complex skills. The piece is made, and when it is done, the person takes what they have made in their hands, touching it and looking at it from many angles. Learning is about to happen.

The woodworker runs fingers over it, feeling its edges and surfaces for smoothness. Holding it to the light and squinting along an edge, the woodworker checks to see if it is straight and true, rechecking dimensions and the fit of every component part.

Then, with these observations in mind, the woodworker reflects about what was done to make the piece, and how to do these things even better next time. The woodworker thinks about the steps – how smoothly a cutting tool did its work, how much material was removed or wasted, whether the piece has a feeling of harmony and rightness – and whether any of these things can be improved. Always, something can be improved.

Based on these observations and reflections, the woodworker tries again, incorporating changes into the work to see if anything will make the work go even better. Over time, the learning continues, often in subtle refinements that a less experienced woodworker might not even notice.

There is an interesting literature about expertise and mastery. One story is that it takes ten thousand hours of deliberate practice to achieve mastery. Learning at this high level happens from experience, reflection, and trying again and again.

Learning that achieves mastery has three related steps. The first step is doing something. The second step is making observations or measurements. The third step is reflecting about how things could have gone even better, and connecting these back to the work in a way that fine-tunes things for the next cycle.

The learning loop

We call these steps the "learning loop."

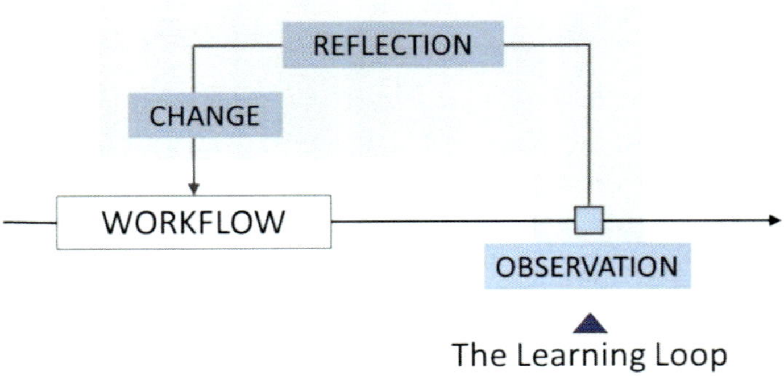

Figure: The learning loop

The elements of the learning loop are 1) a workflow, 2) an observation or measure of the work outcome, and, 3) some process of reflection and change that loops back to the workflow.

If this sounds like a "Plan-Do-Study-Act" improvement cycle, you are right, they are the same. We use the term "learning loop" because this general concept doesn't specify any particular improvement method and is easy to understand from ordinary life experiences.

Methodologies for learning and improvement, such as the Improvement Model, Six Sigma, Lean, TPS and other approaches for improving quality and eliminating waste, are useful. But what matters most is whether the care environment is structured so these methods can make a difference.

Thinking about learning at a team level

Let's take the idea of the learning loop a step farther and consider what it means for an entire care team to learn together.

What is necessary for a team to learn together so it can achieve mastery? We have found it helpful to invite teams to think about learning from the perspective of their entire care team together. Some questions to prompt reflection might be:

- Can you think of any way or place that our entire care team together, including patients and family members, makes observations about how well our care processes are working?

- Can you think of any way or place that our entire care team can intentionally change how we do our work together?

Most teams are puzzled by these questions. Managers are supposed to do these things, aren't they? It is hard for teams to think about learning as something that an entire team does together as a normal part of its work, and to visualize what is necessary for team-level learning to happen well.

People are used to thinking about improvement projects, rather than team-level learning, as a valuable capability.

An infrastructure is necessary for team-level learning

What is necessary for teams to learn at high levels?

Consider the learning loop. The ability to learn as a team requires 1) ways for the team to work together consistently so that learning matters, 2) ways for the entire team to reflect about its work together, and 3) ways that allow observations and reflections of the team to be connected back and change work routines.

So here is the opportunity. In most care environments, measures are rarely available to the care team for observing their work together. Structures are usually not present for reflection as an entire team together, and there are few, if any, pathways available to the team for connecting reflection and change back to their workflows.

Carrying these ideas farther, an infrastructure for team learning can be intentionally introduced into the collaborative care environment by 1) making it possible for a care team to work together consistently, 2) creating opportunities for the care team to meet, observe and reflect together on a regular basis, and 3) creating ways to connect these changes back to the team's work.

Infrastructure for team-level action and reflection

At the beginning of this section we referred to collaborative care environments as "action-reflection learning systems." What does this mean? What is "action" and where does it happen? What is "reflection" and where does it happen? What does "action-reflection learning" have to do with collaborative care?

Think for a moment about a traditional care environment from the perspective of all the people who work there. In most traditional care environments there is plenty of action in the work of daily patient care. People are in motion all the time.

The action may not be very coordinated, and probably happens in "massively parallel" individual work efforts of many people who may not have well-thought-out routines for working as a true team across professions. But, there is plenty of action: orders, calls, charting, rounds, rapid response and code blue calls, admissions, discharges, case management, utilization review, authorizations, in-service meetings, orientations…all of these are the "action" in a traditional care environment.

What about reflection? Does reflection at a team level happen in your care environment? We find that, in general, reflection at a team level doesn't happen in most care environments. It is just not a normal part of the workday for an entire team to meet on a regular basis to reflect about its work together. There is no place, or time, or perceived need to do that. Aren't people too busy to take the time to do that together? I mean, get real here. What are you talking about?

So, the action part doesn't work particularly well because teams aren't consistent, and routines aren't there for doing things together as an entire team. And, the reflection part doesn't happen at all. If that is all true, what about team-level learning? Can it happen in traditional care? What about this idea of practicing and learning over and over to achieve mastery – can this happen? Our answer is, "no" it doesn't happen. Or, maybe, it just barely does. This is the potential, waiting to be unlocked for better care.

So, what about action-reflection learning in collaborative care? Collaborative rounds is the "action" part, with a very clear pattern in which everyone participates. Reflective team meetings are the "reflection" part. Once routines are established for collaborative rounds each day, and reflective team meetings at least weekly or even daily, then the basic infrastructure needed for team learning is in place, and learning accelerates.

Down and In Data

"Down and In Data" means bringing measures of performance and care outcomes "Down and In" to the care team for the purpose of learning. This is in contrast to traditional health care where data is most often reported "Up and Out" to others for purposes of assessment or external accountability.

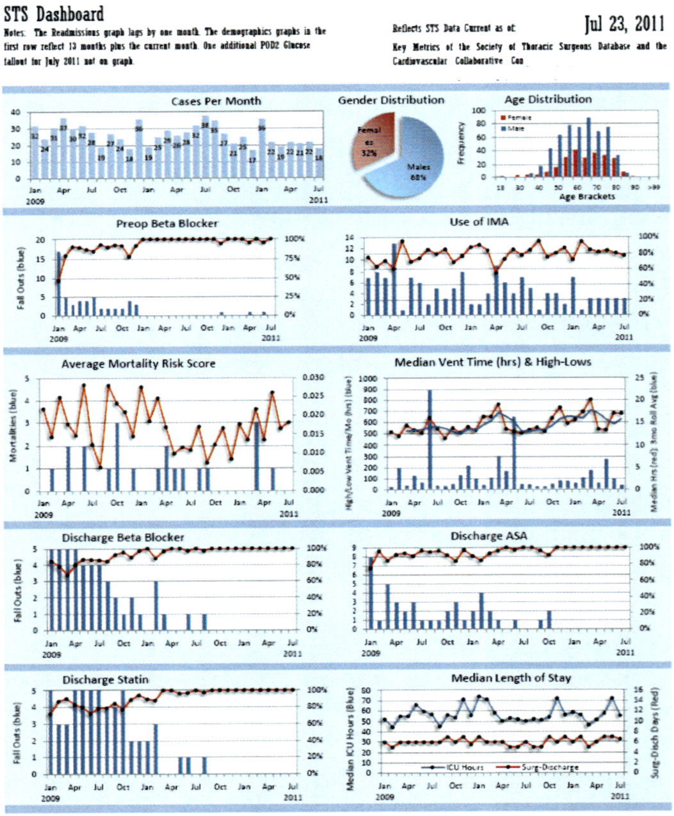

Figure: Down and In Data used by a clinical care team

The figure above is an example of "Down and In Data" developed and used by a collaborative care team. A dashboard of measures was developed by a cardiac surgery team interested in improving its ability to consistently meet all of the quality standards of the Society of Thoracic Surgeons National Database.

At the request of the team, "Down and In Data" was prepared each week by the quality department of the hospital for use in the weekly team meeting. The team used this data as a weekly point of reference as it made changes in its care routines.

If you look carefully at the dashboard, as the team did every week, you are able to see steady improvement over time in measures of preoperative beta blocker use, discharge beta blocker use, discharge statin use, and discharge aspirin use.

These changes were achieved in ongoing cycles of action and reflection informed by the data. Every week in the team meeting, the team reviewed its performance for the week before, discussed the processes behind the data, and made refinements to care routines informed by this ongoing flow of information.

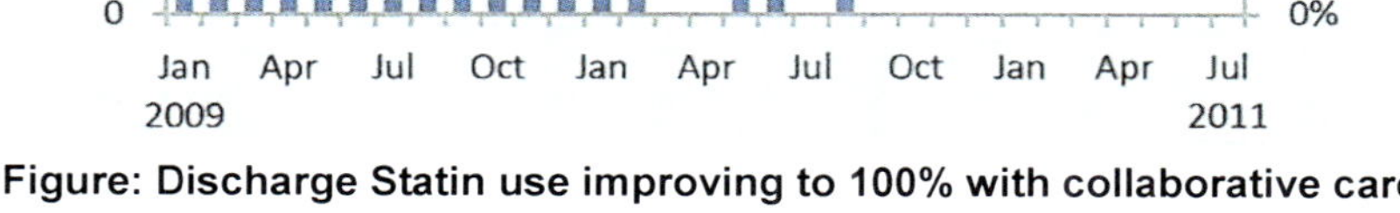

Figure: Discharge Statin use improving to 100% with collaborative care

Notice that certain measures show steady improvement to near-100% reliability. This is illustrated in the chart above of Discharge Statin use, from the lower left corner of the dashboard. Reliability increased to 100%, and fall outs stopped.

The same improvement trends can be seen in the dashboard regarding Preop Beta Blocker, Discharge Beta Blocker, and Discharge Aspirin use. Although standing orders were in place that should have resulted in this care, it was only after collaborative care was instituted that these results were achieved.

Similar use of "Down and In Data" as part of reflective conversations in the weekly team meetings led to revising routines and protocols for many aspects of care, including postoperative blood glucose control, scheduling methods, a preoperative risk assessment protocol, and preoperative evaluations. The weekly team meetings also served as a forum for ongoing development and refinement of other care-related processes and activities, such as a testing clinic and new patient education materials.

"Down and In Data" is most useful when it is reported in a timely manner, for example, reports about last week's care outcomes that are available at this week's team meeting. "Down and In Data" provides the care team with near real-time insights about its performance. Having "Down and In Data" is like connecting the workflows of your team to a vital signs monitor.

Who is present, matters

There is an interesting side story about this use of "Down and In Data." Notice on the previous dashboard that several measures did not change. Examples include Use of IMA (internal mammary artery) and Median Vent Times. The care team members who were meeting weekly included all of the professions caring for cardiac surgery patients, except that five of six cardiac surgeons operating in this unit were not able or willing to participate in the weekly meetings. Changing these measures required changes in the care routines and orders of the surgeons who were not attending the weekly reflection meetings.

The rest of the care team knew that engagement of the surgeons was necessary to make changes in these particular measures. Something else was needed. The team came up with a plan in the weekly meetings in the hope of engaging the surgeons: A quarterly Morbidity and Mortality meeting just for the surgeons. This was planned and initiated by the medical director.

The surgeons did attend the M and M meetings. After these meetings began, the surgeons started to participate in the ongoing improvement efforts, although somewhat reluctantly.

At first, the surgeons didn't want any other professions to attend their meetings, so the medical director, also a surgeon, carried data between the two meetings. Over time, the surgeons became a little more comfortable having others present at the M and M meetings. First the anesthesiologists were able to attend, then perfusionists, and finally nursing and respiratory therapy.

Throughout this time, the weekly team meetings continued for all of the other team members. As the network of connections strengthened and the participation of the surgeons increased, the other outcomes finally began to improve.

There was a definite sense of sadness and resignation among other professions that a separate meeting just for the surgeons was necessary to get everyone working together. People would have gladly changed their meeting time to accommodate the surgeon's schedules. But there was little interest in that from the surgeons.

These are some of the painful realities and power dynamics your team will have to negotiate as you implement collaborative care. However, with persistence over time, significant changes were accomplished and the care environment gradually became more receptive to collaboration.

Summary of things your team can do to use "Down and In Data"

Structures and routines for using "Down and In Data" for the purpose of system learning and improvement can be intentionally implemented. As part of reflective work together, teams can discuss what would be useful to know, and develop ways for collecting this data and making it available to learn about, monitor and improve their collective performance.

- In your reflection meetings you can ask what data about your performance would be useful to know, then develop ways to collect that data and bring it back.
- You can develop a dashboard of key indicators to review and discuss at every weekly team meeting – the data is like having vital signs for your unit.
- You can intentionally use data to learn about your systems and processes of care, and to guide and monitor your efforts to improve your systems.
- You can expect to be surprised by what you see – things are often quite different than you may have thought, and the data will help you see how everyone contributes to your outcomes.
- You can use data to become comfortable looking at and talking about how you are doing as a team, without a sense of blame.
- You can reflect with your team about things you thought you were doing well that actually weren't so good after all – the data lets you see things you may not have recognized before.
- You can reflect with your team about how data helps you stay ahead when people measure you – you will already know what

the measures will show, and can already be working on any concerns.

- You can reflect about whether your mindset is changing – often you can see more clearly where you can do even better, and take pride in trying new things and following the results.

- You can strive to be proactive – your data will let you know about areas where you are doing really well, and know about any concerns early so you can make intentional changes.

- You can reflect with your team about what you took for granted in the past – some teams say they were driving in the dark without headlights but didn't know it – the lights are on now.

GLITCH Process

A GLITCH process is a way of monitoring and improving the performance of a care system in a different way than using measures. The term GLITCH was first used in the Concord collaborative care program. It was a deliberate word choice intended to minimize the sense of blame or shame that so often is felt in health care when things don't go right. The term GLITCH was intended to help the team talk openly about things that did not go right in a constructive and receptive way, without a sense that someone had done something wrong.

Even with this understanding, there was still a lingering sense of failure and shame about GLITCHes. After using the term GLITCH for several months, a pharmacist on the team wanted to change that perception. One day he called the team together. He said that he had figured out what GLITCH stands for. He wrote the letters G-L-I-T-C-H on the board and said, "GLITCH means 'Gathering Little Insights That Can Help'."

With this added definition the word GLITCH became the vehicle it was intended to be. From that day forward, people were almost always able to identify GLITCHes with interest and curiosity rather than a sense of failure. Whenever something didn't go as expected, the word GLITCH helped the team see that particular event as an opportunity to talk about how their system of care system might be changed to make the GLITCH go away.

This is how a GLITCH process can work. With every activity that the team does while caring for patients, build in a few moments to ask each other, the patient, and family members to think back about the care with this question: "Is there anything that could have happened differently or better?" If this question is asked and time is given for people to think about the question, you will almost always find a few things that didn't go exactly right.

Some of the things identified as GLITCHes are glaring problems, and many more are minor concerns. But almost all GLITCHes represent opportunities for improving your system of care. A seemingly minor event might have underlying roots that could surface in more serious ways. Even things that are not perceived as serious but that take time and attention away from other care activities can have important benefits when these are recognized and redesigned at a root level.

Take time to ask about GLITCHes during each patient encounter and after every procedure or other activity, then note any GLITCHes and talk about them at the next weekly team meeting. You will be surprised how this helps your team identify things that can be steadily improved in your care environment.

At first, care teams may be reluctant to talk openly about GLITCHes, especially in front of patients and families. Leadership modeling that explores GLITCHes transparently with the team, including patients and families, is helpful for having people reconsider this orientation. Over a few months of doing this, it will become routine to talk about these things together.

Below are examples of some actual GLITCHes:

"Medication orders are being faxed to food service instead of to the pharmacy"
-moved the speed dial buttons on the phone so they were at opposite corners

"The light in the shower is dim"
-installed a brighter bulb in the shower

"We gave one patient's insulin to a different patient"
-label printer was broken, tests were mislabeled. Back up printer ordered

"We were told that the doctor would talk to us after surgery but he came two hours later"
-chaplain will check on each patient and keep in touch with the surgeon

"Wish we could have been with our mother during shift change"
-long conversation resulting in new open visiting hour policy

"We meant to give Lasix but forgot to put in the order"
-changed routine so orders are written in real time on rounds rather than later

"The sterile wrap on the instrument tray wasn't completely sealed"
-new processing method developed by Central Supply

"The patient had a latex allergy but we didn't know it"
-computer display changed to always show latex allergy

"We didn't know the patient was a Jehovah's Witness until the day he came for surgery"
-new proactive protocol developed for Jehovah's Witness patients

"When we put a brighter light in the shower we could see mold there"
-Oh my! new cleaning routines instituted for shower rooms

Figure: Examples of actual GLITCHes and improvements made

As part of this learning, consider asking patients and family members how it felt to have GLITCHes discussed. You will learn that one of the greatest fears of patients and families is that things are being hidden from them. As patients and families see that the care team is actively seeking and openly discussing these kinds of events and situations, a notably new level of trust develops.

To collect GLITCHes during procedures, it is helpful to keep a blank sheet of paper labeled "GLITCH – No Blame" in a convenient place where the procedure is being done. As the operation or procedure proceeds, when things don't go quite right, as they inevitably will, simply note those things on the GLITCH sheet. At the end of the procedure, take a moment to review the GLITCHes and ask if there is anything else that should be added or mentioned. Then, at the next team meeting, discuss the GLITCHes as part of the meeting.

As unexpected events come to your attention, even if they are not considered a safety event, note them as a GLITCH. We suggest not making any determination of whether a GLITCH is major or minor. Things that look minor might be recognized as part of a larger pattern when discussed in the weekly system meetings. An important feature of recording GLITCHes is making a deliberate effort not to identify a GLITCH in any particular way, for example as a 'safety concern' or a 'quality concern' because these are emotionally laden terms. Simply take note of things as GLITCHes, and remind people that you want to find every GLITCH they experienced so you can make your systems better.

Asking about GLITCHes during rounds invites everyone present to think about whether anything could have gone better in the patient's care. A GLITCH might also be positive – a serendipitous discovery of a potentially beneficial unexpected event. This invitation to consider GLITCHes opens a space for every person's sense of what is notable as a GLITCH, which you will find varies with personal and professional experience, education, training, and many other perceptions.

You will be surprised at the conversations that are generated and the bottleneck of unresolved GLITCHes that your team will begin to uncover. As you discuss and improve the underlying system causes for your GLITCHes, you will begin to experience benefits. Things will begin to go more smoothly in the day-to-day routines of care, your team will begin to have more time because long-standing work arounds are no longer needed, and there will be a growing sense of accomplishment and capability that comes from knowing that you can change things. You will be surprised when you review your GLITCHes later at how much has changed from this work.

Over time, as the self-awareness of the collaborative team grows and its identity strengthens through shared learning, a natural curiosity will arise that will accelerate learning even more.

Type 1 and Type 2 problem solving

Based on the work of Anita Tucker, who observed nurses solving problems during their shifts for her PhD dissertation research, nurses solved problems in two ways during their work of caring for patients. "First order" or Type 1 problem solving is doing something that solves an immediate concern but doesn't change underlying root causes of the problem. "Second order" or Type 2 problem solving addresses the situation at a root level.

Anita found that almost all (93%) of the problem solving by nurses was Type 1, resolving a problem for the moment but doing nothing to prevent it from happening again. An additional 6% of the problems solving she observed was Type 1, but a supervisor was notified. Just 1% of the problem solving she observed involved creating Type 2 root level solutions.

We believe that Type 1 problem solving is the norm in traditional care, because people working on the front lines of health care don't have a way of doing anything else. We have found that using these terms of Type 1 and Type 2 problem solving gives people a language for thinking about their work and their care environment in a way that awakens curiosity and awareness.

The achievement of reliability and resilience in collaborative care requires a shift from Type 1 to Type 2 problem solving. Unresolved system problems are pervasive in traditional health care environments. Much of the daily effort of care team members is absorbed by Type 1 problem-solving activities. In traditional health care, there is a resignation to this as an unpleasant but necessary fact of life. There is little opportunity for front line team members, patients, or family members to do anything about the daily system frustrations that are encountered.

In collaborative care, the nature of care incorporates ongoing cycles of action and reflection as an intentional part of the normal work of the care team. An infrastructure is intentionally established for eliciting system concerns, reflecting about them, and responding to them at a collective level in Type 2 ways.

This integration of system monitoring and improvement into daily work routines makes it possible for care teams to continuously refine their work context, making work progressively easier and more effective. It also holds the care team in a state of continuous mindfulness about the way that care happens, and how it can become even better. This self-aware, engaged perspective not only improves reliability, it helps to build resilience.

Summary of things your team can do to develop a GLITCH process

Structures and routines can be intentionally implemented for continuously testing and refining systems. A GLITCH process begins by asking about GLITCHes – anything that happened unexpectedly or that could have gone better. Routines can be developed for asking about GLITCHes and considering them in reflective team meetings.

- You can develop routines for asking about GLITCHes as part of everything you do, including on rounds and after other activities such as operations and procedures.

- You can learn to be comfortable asking about GLITCHes – at first, people may be embarrassed or worried, but with time it becomes much easier, and patients actually like it.

- You can record GLITCHes as you identify them, and bring them to your system meetings to discuss among your team and hopefully resolve at a root cause level.

- You can encourage your team to see GLITCHes as opportunities for system improvement that are inevitable in any system, not as failures or mistakes that requires blame or criticism.

- You can help people realize that not every GLITCH can be resolved right away. Sometimes you won't know what to do differently – trend those to see if they happen again.

- Intentionally, don't decide if a GLITCH is major or minor – it is surprising what turns out to matter. Treat everything as important if it is something that didn't go as you expected.

- You can help your team recognize how often things didn't go the way you wanted in the past, yet those things were just tolerated – with GLITCHes you are able to identify system problems and resolve them.

- You can encourage your team to talk about Type 1 and Type 2 problem solving – Type 1 is smoothing over a

GLITCH, while Type 2 is fixing it at a root level, which often your team will be able to do by working together.

- You can help people to expect surprises from GLITCHes – often they show things you wouldn't have known about any other way.

- You can keep a record of your GLITCHes and the changes you make – otherwise you may forget how much progress you have made. Those records of improvement will help you get organizational support for your work.

The Benefits of Team Learning

The importance of establishing an infrastructure for team learning cannot be overstated. The daily collaborative care routines will take a while to have running smoothly, but eventually people will not want to work any other way. The weekly team meetings give people a chance to sit down and consider care systems together, and begin to learn together. Almost any hoped-for change in routines involves many members of the care team.

With an opportunity for everyone to meet, talk, reflect, plan, and monitor changes together, the work of making thoughtful changes in care routines has a central home. It will become very comfortable for your team to work and learn like this. People will enjoy their work more, and relationships between people will become more meaningful. Your care outcomes will also improve.

A story is helpful for illustrating the benefits of team learning in this regard. The cardiac surgery team at Concord Hospital was working to reduce the length of time patients were on a ventilator before removal of the breathing tube after cardiac operations. Because the entire care team had a routine of meeting weekly, the anesthesiologists, surgeons, nurses, pharmacists, and respiratory therapists who needed to work together to reduce ventilator times were able each week to discuss their progress and make continual refinements of their work routines together.

The hospital was part of a regional quality network. Programs at the other hospitals in the network were also trying to decrease ventilator times.

An important difference between programs was the weekly reflective team meetings of the collaborative program, which provided a regular opportunity for the collaborative care team to meet and learn together. The other programs did not have this infrastructure for collaborative learning.

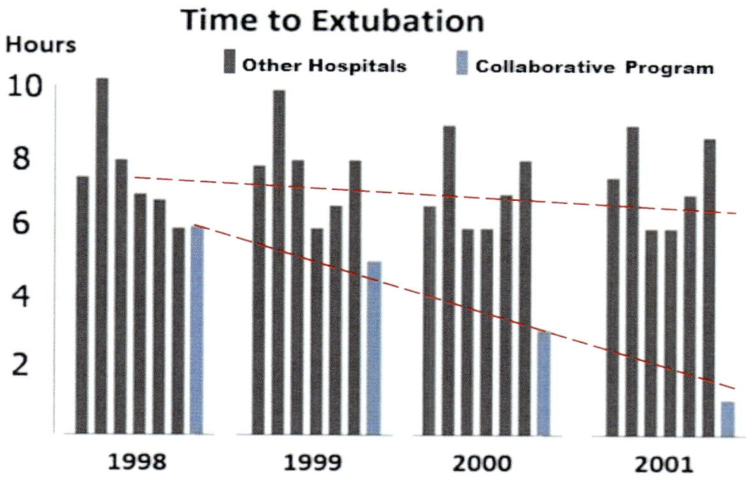

Figure: Ability to change established routines is enhanced

Over several years the team with the weekly team learning infrastructure was able to decrease the average ventilator time from nearly six hours to 45 minutes. The other hospitals made progress, too, but much less than the progress achieved in the collaborative program, as shown in the figure above.

Evolution of the Collaborative Care Environment

The figure below illustrates the growth of reliability and resilience in care teams. The figure illustrates that reliability and resilience emerge from interactions, reflection, and team-level learning in addition to the development of individual skills.

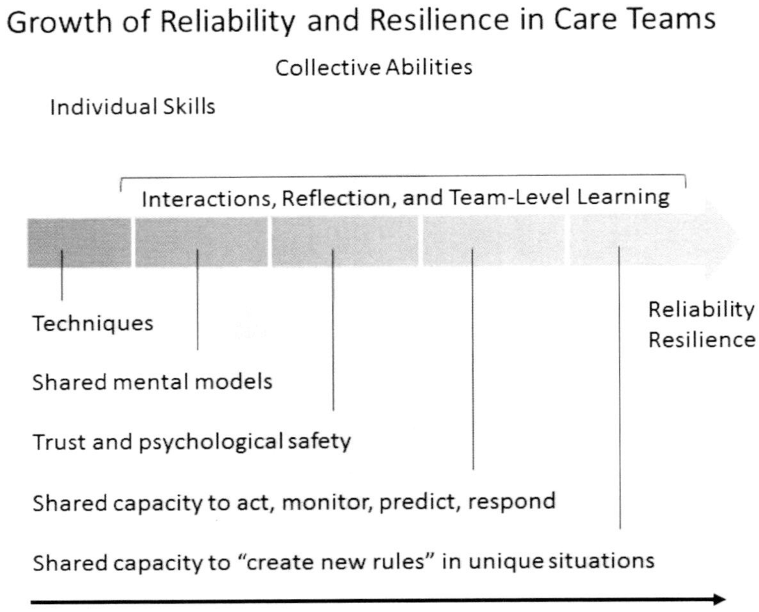

Figure: Social origins of reliability and resilience

Although basic techniques for collaborative care can be taught through teamwork training, deeper attributes of reliability and resilience are collective abilities of the care team that go beyond individual teamwork skills. These collective capabilities grow and develop through ongoing social interactions of the care team when conditions in the local care environment support consistent interactions, shared reflection, and team-level learning.

Achieving Reliability and Resilience

This section considers how reliability and resilience develop in collaborative care. These mastery-level attributes are properties of social fields that develop because of the connections that exist, and the team-level learning and ongoing system refinements that are enabled, in collaborative care environments.

Reliability and resilience are topics of richly-evolving scholarship in safety science. Reliability and resilience are complementary and distinct attributes of exceptional teams and organizations. The distinctions between reliability and resilience concern the nature of the situations that teams inevitably face.

Let's first consider reliability. There are many things that a health care team experiences and does every day that are routine. An important aspect of reliability that develops in collaborative care environments is being able to care for patients in routine situations in consistent and effective ways, every time.

Often in health care, situations are not routine. Many of the non-routine situations that a care team encounters happen frequently enough that planned responses can be developed and refined. An example might be fetal distress requiring a Caesarian section. This is not normal and can be serious, but responses can be planned and utilized that will greatly improve the likelihood of a good outcome. We call these kinds of situations "normally abnormal." An important aspect of reliability in collaborative care is being able to recognize and respond to "normally abnormal" situations in effective ways through team-level learning.

An additional dimension of reliability is the ability to monitor these "normally abnormal" events, learn from them, and make system changes so they are recognized earlier, become less frequent, and eventually can be prevented altogether.

Sometimes, though, care teams encounter situations that are abnormal in ways they have never experienced before, and that could not have been predicted, mitigated, or prevented based on prior events. We call these kinds of situations "abnormally abnormal." These kinds of events may be so far outside of prior experience that no previously developed response can be applied with certainty, and unpredictable enough that no preventative improvement strategy could have been applied beforehand.

In these "abnormally abnormal" situations the care team is operating in an area of uncertainty that calls for a different kind of capability. Highly functioning collaborative care teams are able to recognize when a situation has become "abnormally abnormal," and respond as effectively at these times as they do when things are routine or "normally abnormal." One member of a collaborative care team said, "We don't know exactly what we will do in those situations, but we have developed ways of working really well together, so we can figure something out." That is resilience.

Researchers who study and write about resilience emphasize the importance of human actions in resilient systems. When situations move past the known and resilience is required, the responses of people, rather than technology, is what usually makes the difference. The development of resilience is one of the highest levels of evolution of the collaborative care environment.

Resilience is more than flexibility. Responding effectively in the face of something entirely unexpected requires improvisation and innovation, finding ways despite uncertainty to come up with a path forward that may never have been tried before.

One dimension of resilience concerns the medical and technical care of the patient. In well-functioning collaborative settings, the entire care team is working together in ways that make routine medical care second nature. This allows very early detection of departures from routines. Also, in well-functioning collaborative care, ideas, insights and actions are able to emerge that were not in the mind of anyone when the conversation began.

Resilience in "abnormally abnormal" situations

During our research about collaborative care we have observed care team interactions that demonstrated resilience, and others that did not. In this section we will describe an example of each. These descriptions are from debriefings conducted by Cindy Dominguez, a cognitive scientist and member of our research team. Both happened with patients on the same cardiac surgery service. However, one took place in an ICU setting where people worked closely together on a regular basis, and the other took place on a postoperative floor where there was a less well-developed collaborative care environment.

The first episode involved high blood glucose levels that did not respond to usual methods of treatment. In the care of cardiac surgery patients, blood glucose levels often require treatment with a continuous infusion of intravenous insulin. This is a common, "normally abnormal" pattern after heart surgery, for which a treatment protocol had been developed by this care team.

During the care of a particular patient, the insulin infusion protocol did not work as expected. When the bedside nurse started the insulin protocol, the blood glucose level kept going up instead of stabilizing. The nurse increased the insulin infusion rate to progressively higher levels, and checked the blood glucose more frequently, yet the level continued to increase. The nurse had never seen this response before and decided to consult more experienced nurses. Together they checked the lines and pumps. Word spread quickly through the unit about the situation. The nurses agreed they had not seen a blood glucose response like this before on their protocol. The nurse manager was contacted.

Thirty minutes later, after multiple adjustments had been made, the blood glucose level was still not responding. By then several nurses were on Google, researching possible explanations and offering help. The patient's nurse began seeking information outside of the unit. He asked the hospital pharmacist if there was a maximum dose of insulin that could be given, and for suggestions about what should be done. The pharmacist sent up a new bag of insulin. All tubing was changed out. Glucose levels were checked by an alternate lab method.

By 0430 the nurse called the medical director of the unit, giving him an update and asking his advice. The medical director said that he had never seen this before either, and suggested a maximum infusion rate and continued observation. He offered to come see the patient, but the nurse felt this was not necessary for the time being. At 0530, the nurse called the patient's surgeon to be sure he was informed. At 0700, just at the shift-to-shift handover, the blood glucose level finally began dropping. The night nurse updated the day nurse, who stayed at the bedside adjusting the insulin until the patient was stable. A cause for the high levels was never identified. The patient eventually did well.

During a critical incident debriefing led by Cindy to map how the team made decisions together, the pharmacist, medical director, other nurses, and the nurse manager described what they did to support the bedside nurse during the care of this patient – researching, running down leads, working to understand the issue. Was there a bad batch of insulin? No... Research on insulin resistance? No, only found in rat studies..., etc. The nurse caring for the patient said he felt supported throughout the event, even though no one was completely sure what was happening.

Summarizing the reflections from the debriefing, Cindy described the pattern of response of this team as a "Cocoon Model." The nurse and the patient were enveloped in a cocoon of support by a cohesive team of professionals acting in concert.

During this episode, the bedside nurse recognized that the situation was abnormal in a way he had not experienced before. Others confirmed this. The nurse asked for advice and people responded, providing support proactively and remaining informed and connected, prepared to do even more if needed.

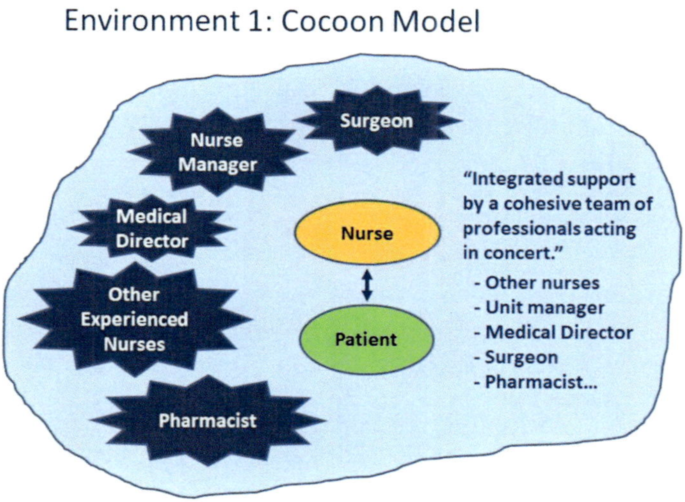

Figure: "Cocoon Model" of integrated support – Cindy Dominguez

In contrast to this event, a different nurse and patient had a more difficult experience in the setting of the postoperative floor. A patient was recovering after bypass surgery, but had a medical condition called myasthenia gravis which can cause weakness and difficulty breathing. It is an uncommon condition that many people on the care team had not seen before, at least not in patients after heart surgery. Having a postoperative heart patient with myasthenia gravis was well outside their usual experience.

After an unremarkable initial postoperative course, the patient began not feeling well early one morning, which was recognized by his nurse. However, despite multiple telephone calls to others, the actual cause of the patient's condition was not identified until much later in the day, when the patient had a near respiratory arrest requiring placement of a breathing tube and transfer back to the intensive care unit.

The confusion and frustration of this care team is evident in transcripts from a debriefing that Cindy conducted:

Nurse: *"I was frustrated all day long. From 0730 to 0930 the patient is telling me he just doesn't feel right. I am concerned, even though the O2 saturation is fine."*

Nurse practitioner: *"The bedside nurse just told me she had a bad feeling and something just was not right with him and so we went in together and assessed him at 0930. The surgeon showed up and I told him what was going on. He said the patient just needs to walk a bit more in the hall."*

Nurse: *"I called the cardiologist's assistant and said I'd like to have a chest x-ray and she said no, he had an x-ray yesterday. She said call the radiologist and let me know what you see."*

Nurse practitioner: *"In between 1000 and 1100 I went into the patient's room and the bedside nurse was frustrated – she said, 'no one is listening to me and taking me seriously. They don't believe me…'*

Nurse: *"At 1030 another RT said, "I am concerned about your patient." I said, 'Would you call the cardiology PA?' The RT called the cardiology PA, who ordered a blood gas and gave me an order for an EKG. EKG came around 1045, and it was normal sinus rhythm. The cardiologist called me and said 'call me directly if you need anything else' – I got the sense he was concerned. I would have liked to hear him say, 'I will be there to see him shortly,' or 'let's get him transferred.'*

Nurse: *"Around noon we got the x-ray and he had bilateral pleural effusions. The assistant said we're not going to worry about it – it's better than yesterday. She told me to call the neurologist back on the case because she didn't think it was cardiac related. The patient was telling the neurologist, through labored breathing, what he was experiencing. She said she didn't think it was typical myasthenia gravis. She went to the doc box and wrote an order for an extra med for myasthenia, though. Within an hour the patient was intubated and in the ICU."*

Respiratory Therapist: *"I didn't know the patient had a history of myasthenia…"*

Nurse Manager: *"It took from about 9 in the morning when she first raised the bell, until 4 pm that afternoon, for, really, the right intervention to have occurred."*

Like the first episode, this care team was experiencing a situation that was "abnormally abnormal." However, unlike the first episode, this care team was not able to account for the puzzling condition of the patient and respond outside of usual patterns. Even though individual people felt uncomfortable, including the patient's nurse, the team was not able to recognize that the situation was outside of usual routines, and didn't develop alternative responses that might have prevented the near arrest.

It is important to emphasize that everyone involved in the care of this patient meant well, and that the individual skills of the care team members are not the focus of this discussion. Rather, the emphasis is that a care team in one environment was able to quickly move into a resilience mode, whereas another group of people in a different part of the care environment was not.

Summarizing the reflections from the debriefing of the second episode, Cindy described the pattern of response of this team as a "Constellation of Stars." The nurse and the patient were on their own, dependent upon multiple inquiries by the nurse, and upon the responses of multiple providers who were not working from a collaborative perspective.

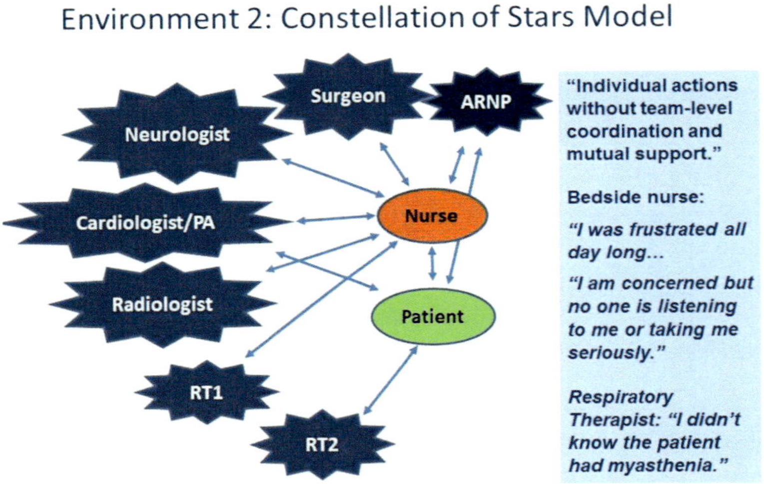

Figure: "Constellation of Stars Model" – Cindy Dominguez

During this episode, the bedside nurse recognized that the situation was abnormal, but could not activate the other providers in a timely or coordinated way. We believe the difference between episodes is largely explained by the connections and patterns of interactions that were quite different between the two environments. In the ICU setting, people knew each other well, were used to working together, and had plenty of practice responding to many kinds of events as a team. In the floor setting, people were mostly doing individual tasks separately from one another. When the need for resilience arose, the people in the floor environment simply did not have those resources and connections to draw from.

Stories of resilience and healing

The experiences of patients and family members undergoing medical care can be life altering. Resilience is necessary for patients and families who have to go through these experiences and somehow emerge intact on the other side. Usually this kind of resilience comes from human connections. Simply knowing that others are present and care, can be a remarkable source of mutual strength and healing.

There is a story that illustrates this healing kind of resilience. A patient was in the intensive care unit, critically ill on a ventilator. A day after her breathing tube was removed, she said to the team during rounds, "I don't ever give up. That's who I am." As the team listened, she told them about her four children. She had lost custody of them after an unsuccessful marriage during a difficult time in her life. She said that she was working to win their love and respect back, one child at a time. She said she had fully reconnected with two children and her grandchildren, and was having increasing contact with the other two children.

On rounds several days later, with the patient out of the intensive care unit, one of the care team members thanked her for her story about never giving up and told her what an impact her story made on the team. He said, "I just wanted you to know that we see you." Another person said, "Your story about not giving up made us not want to give up on you, either."

A different patient had a deep-seated fear of having anything over her mouth or face. She had grown up in Germany during World War II. Her fear was from memories of air raids she had experienced every night as a little girl. Her mother had been killed in one of the air raids. Her stories touched the hearts of the care team. They patiently and lovingly held her in their arms as she recovered from anesthesia. The next day the patient thanked the care team for all they did. Her nurse said, "My goal is to spend every minute I can with you. You make *my* heart happy."

These stories are about the human connections that are possible in collaborative environments, and what they produce. Every interaction between these patients and the other members of the care team was warmer, richer, and wiser because of these experiences and the connections they established. The connections that develop over time among people in collaborative care environments are resources that can be drawn from later. They promote healing in many ways. Resilience grows from this.

Reliability, resilience, and social fields

The literature on resilience emphasizes four primary abilities of the resilient team or organization: *responding, learning, anticipating, and monitoring*. The Social Field Model of Collaborative Care encompasses these abilities and adds *engagement with patients and families, the ability to invite and welcome, emergence, and aliveness (of the human spirit).*

The emergence of reliability and resilience in collaborative care is an expression of the full development of a collaborative social field. Reliability and resilience are social accomplishments that advance the care team far beyond individual capabilities. Fully developed collaborative care allows every dimension of reliability and resilience, human and technical, to flourish.

Good for the human spirit

A marker of the emergence of reliability and resilience is a strong sense of meaning and purpose that exceptional teams experience in their daily work.

In the literature about resilience, it is emphasized that human actions are at the core of resilience. As we have reflected about resilience as it manifests in collaborative care, it is clear to us that human connections between people create a sense of aliveness of the human spirit that is closely linked with resilience. People "carry each other" across the uncertainties, lifting each other up with knowledge, dignity, comfort and care.

The infrastructure for team learning in highly evolved collaborative care environments makes it possible for people to be active participants in care at two levels – able to participate in the care of each patient in meaningful ways, and able to make intentional changes to improve the functioning of their own care environment. This is true for professional care team members, and also for patients and family members. This connection between learning, engagement, impact, and aliveness of the human spirit is at the heart of collaborative care.

We believe that reliability and resilience will increasingly be understood as flowing from deep connections among people and with their work. This sense of connectedness, and the sense of meaning that flows from it, is a primary motivating force in collaborative care. This is important for technical reliability and resilience, and especially important for the resilience of healing.

In collaborative care, connection-based reliability and resilience are reciprocal among all involved. They are resources that grow in a positive spiral of increasing strength, capability and benefit for everyone who is able to participate in their co-creation.

PART SIX

SUSTAINING

- Is Collaborative Care Right for Your Organization?
- Simulation and Interprofessional Education
- Becoming a Model for Others

Is Collaborative Care Right for Your Organization?

The goal of this section is to provoke thought about sustainability. By sustainability we mean ways that a collaborative environment can have a natural home in a setting that recognizes its value, furthers its development, and identifies with its success.

For those of us who believe in collaborative care and treasure its beauty and benefits, this section is difficult and bittersweet to write. The other sections of the Field Guide are written based on success. We are certain from extensive experience that the recommendations they contain will guide you well. This section is written based on failures. We are not certain yet about the recommendations this section contains, because we haven't yet fully solved the challenges of sustainability.

We think from our experience that the keys to sustainability have to do with connections between the local care environment and its larger organizational context. Whereas implementing collaborative care depends on structures and social preconditions at the local team level, sustaining collaborative care depends on the nature of the contexts in which the local environment exists and how well the local environment connects to the larger organization and beyond.

Although health care happens at a front line level, very few health care organizations are constituted so simply. Instead, they are complex – with divisions, departments, leadership levels, and other more complex forms of organizational design. The collaborative care environment at a local level must connect well within this larger organizational context if it is to survive and thrive.

Also, there are many powerful contexts that organizations function within that affect the collaborative environment. These include larger organizational structures, such as health systems, and an array of other entities and shaping forces such as payment policies, accreditation processes, education standards, training and certification standards, and general societal expectations.

In our experience, most failures of collaborative care happen after initially successful implementation efforts, and are related to misalignment between the non-hierarchical, intentionally generative nature of collaborative care and the expectations of existing organizational structures and management methods of most traditional health care organizations.

Although successful implementation and sustainability of collaborative care can happen in traditional organizational structures, you may wish to consider how well collaborative care will fit in your present organizational culture. It is clear to us that the next frontier of collaborative care is organizational redesign.

Some health care organizations are deciding that traditional operating models must be reconfigured to meet increasing requirements for reliability, resilience, responsiveness, and innovation. Organizations exploring innovative management models designed to achieve these goals may be an ideal supportive home for collaborative care. A good test is the question: Does the way our organization is structured and led match the structures and leadership methods required at a local level for the emergence of collaborative care?

A guiding principle is that that there should be a fractal-like resonance between the organizational structures that surround the collaborative care initiative, and the front line care environment itself. In other words, the nature of your organization needs to match the nature of the desired collaborative care environment for collaborative care to be successful and sustainable.

Organizational characteristics supporting successful implementation and sustainability of collaborative care

We have come to believe there are certain characteristics at a leadership and organizational level that are helpful for successfully implementing and sustaining collaborative care.

These are:

- commitment to honesty and full disclosure
- willingness to distribute power and share information
- patience and courage to intentionally commit significant resources in anticipation of long term benefits
- tolerance for ambiguity, and acceptance that progress will be unpredictable
- organizational and political will to absorb organizational and political distress that will inevitably arise at various times during the implementation process
- determination to achieve exceptional performance over and beyond meeting external standards or benchmarks
- priority of service mission over other goals

It is important to recognize that collaborative care needs to be led and supported organizationally in ways that often differ from traditional administrative approaches in many health care organizations. Collaborative care depends upon the emergence of a certain "state of being" within the care team that requires administrative and leadership support. This state of being is characterized by certain attributes that need to have a comfortable home and resonance within the authorizing organizational context.

These include:

- a high degree of psychological safety
- comfort participating in self-directed processes
- focus on meaning and advocacy over following rules
- recognition of the essential role of engagement and participation in care, decision making, and healing
- highly developed listening skills concerning the needs, thoughts, and suggestions of other team members, including patients and family members
- nuanced awareness of usual patterns of care and patient course, combined with highly developed ability to detect and respond to departures from patterns
- integral use of simple processes and metrics for monitoring and improving clinical systems

Each of these has a parallel at an organizational level. The likelihood of sustainability of a collaborative initiative depends on whether the organization values and exemplifies this way of being.

Collaborative care is "enabled from above, and built from below." This supports the insights of Vogus and Singer that high reliability organizations are "enabled" through the advocacy and support of organizational leaders, and "enacted" (built) and "elaborated" (developed) by the day-to-day actions and evolving beliefs of care team members, patients, and family members.

A crucial insight and distinction from traditional practice is that people must be "invited into" collaborative care. Its nature requires this. It is likely that collaborative care will be a good fit in your organization if leaders and managers are trying to do things in ways that respectfully invite and engage all participants in developing goals and ways of achieving goals, and of self-monitoring and refining performance in ways that flow from front line teams to senior leaders and then throughout the organization.

If, however, and more likely, leaders in your organization make decisions centrally, and if performance goals are driven by leaders and managers who hold others accountable for achieving them, collaborative care will be harder to enact and sustain.

An inherent tension

Surprising fault lines can develop between the collaborative environment and its organizational context. There may be an inherent tension between what a collaborative unit naturally evolves to become, and what traditional organizations expect a care unit and its leadership should be like. It may seem at first to leaders that collaborative care is a good idea, but as the realities of what collaborative care means in terms of engagement and self-determination play out, the unit may be increasingly perceived as out of alignment with organizational expectations.

As collaborative care takes root, the local hierarchy at the unit level will flatten, and control will become much more distributed. At the center of the care process, control will increasingly flow away from traditional leaders and processes to the collaborative team itself, including patients and families, who are now functioning in a different way with less hierarchy and control. Organizational policies and procedures may increasingly be seen as burdensome and restrictive in comparison to the highly responsive, locally generated modes of the awakening group.

In general, there is initial excitement at the level of senior management about the idea of collaborative care and the benefits that could come from better coordination, communication, and teamwork at a front-line level. At first, there is likely to be organizational support for these kinds of transformational activities. However, as the collaborative team becomes more capable, and increasing levels of functional autonomy develop, the stresses that these changes induce throughout the organization may become significant.

Stressful for leaders and managers

Let's consider why this might happen. In traditional health care organizations, the flow of ideas and authority often happens in a directive way. Goals are established, and policies and procedures are developed and directed into the organization, from senior leaders to directors to managers and finally to the front line staff. Processes are established, staffing grids are developed, budgets are prepared, and all of this is enacted through an accountability structure of reporting relationships.

Also, the requests made of the organization to achieve co-location, consistent staffing, and regular reflection time may be perceived as particularly troubling and too far outside of the norm.

Imagine in this context that an increasingly autonomous collaborative front-line care environment is successfully established and begins to outperform every other unit in the organization. The unit by its new nature does not follow rules, it makes them. Managers and leaders who view their job as directing people may be surprised and puzzled by this autonomy that infringes on their usual feelings of responsibility and control.

Also, imagine that the changes at the front line level do cause some problems locally. There will always be some degree of unhappiness with any change. It is inevitable that the changes of collaborative care will disturb some established norms and patterns, which will cause distress for at least a few people. In any good organization this distress will be recognized and transmitted upward through leadership channels. If the upper-level leaders are functioning in usual ways, they are likely to watch this closely, so they can proactively take actions to resolve any concerns.

In fact, the unit is developing its own ability to manage the distress of change through local social means. But frequently, the response of the organization is out of phase and behind the evolving capabilities of the front line unit. The unit may appear to be struggling from a traditional perspective, when in fact, it is just beginning to function at its best in a new autonomous way.

Unless there is a good understanding of what is actually happening at the front line level, and, particularly, if the collaborative care initiative has not yet made a visible impact in measurable quality or satisfaction outcomes, a conclusion may be reached that the new initiative is causing too much distress and must be brought under better control.

Front line teams and hospital departments

An interesting illustration of the tensions that can develop between a collaborative front line care environment and traditional hospital departments occurred when a collaborative team created its own patient satisfaction survey. Within a short time, the survey was designed, implemented, and put to use. It was given to patients and families by bedside nurses and discussed several days later at the weekly team meetings. There was excitement as this new process began to generate new insights.

Several weeks after the survey was instituted, a message was received from the hospital administration: "No surveys are to be done of patient satisfaction unless formally approved by the quality department." A representative from the quality department came to the weekly team meeting to tell the team about all the mistakes being made according to hospital policies in the work they were doing. The interaction was emotionally devastating for the care team, and the entire process ended.

A similar story with a different outcome concerned an initiative to develop a GLITCH process as described in an earlier section of this guide. After several weeks developing the process, it became routine that 3 to 5 GLITCHes were being identified each day about processes or systems that did not work as intended or that needed to be in place and were not. The front-line GLITCH process was quickly producing a steady stream of insights about things that could be made even better in the care environment.

Soon, however, a communication came from the hospital administration. The team was informed that they must use an electronic process which was in place for entering these concerns rather than the GLITCH process they had developed. They were told there was a form that had to be filed online, and an official process must be followed to document and respond to these concerns. The team was assured that the process was easy to use and would result in improvement at an organizational level.

An effort was made to utilize both the new process and the official one, and to compare their effectiveness. Using the front-line methods, it took only a few seconds to ask about and record any GLITCHes as these were identified. It took nearly 5 minutes to log onto the hospital website, find the right page, and complete the online form in the extensive detail required by the hospital system.

The care team asked what became of the forms they submitted on line, because no feedback was ever returned to them. The forms were eventually found, printed out and unread, in stacks on the desk of a single person in the quality office. Over time, the team quietly kept doing its own GLITCH identification, and stopped doing the official process.

These examples are not intended to be critical. They are meant simply to highlight the difference between locally-generated collaborative efforts and the departmentally-based systems in most health care organizations. The point is that these two approaches, while potentially compatible, can easily come in conflict without careful attention to connecting them together. The important work of connecting front line efforts with those of the larger organization can carry stresses of emotion, power, and worry about loss of control in both directions. Good connections can be achieved, but creating them requires thoughtful attention.

Puzzling and stressful for practitioners, too

Similarly, collaborative care often produces initial distress among physicians and other care providers with authority and power in traditional health care. A collaborative model does not match these traditional expectations.

As the front line environment changes to a more level power structure, and attention begins to be focused more on the human experience of everyone involved, a reorienting of priorities starts to occur in front line care. This has the tendency of reducing the primacy of traditional medical aspects of care, and increasing emphasis on human aspects of care and the care experience.

These changes can be disconcerting and may even seem inappropriate from the perspective of physicians and others who have been trained to provide care under their direct control. There are likely to be physicians who will not recognize the value and benefits of collaborative care, and, in fact, may see collaborative care as a threat or barrier to getting their work done effectively and efficiently.

A topic for discussion by your team in your weekly meetings is how your team will respond when these kinds of tensions and events arise with physicians and with other areas and leaders in your organization. We encourage you to talk respectfully yet openly about these situations, and discuss ways that your team can manage them in productive ways.

Two stories help to illustrate the need for this.

During one of our research observations, a collaborative care team we were observing was functioning at a remarkably high level. An enjoyable conversation was happening between the patient, family members, and professional members of the care team. Laughter was frequent, and plans were being jointly developed and recorded on the goal board.

In the middle of that conversation, a physician who had not been part of a collaborative care process entered the room. He walked directly to the patient, who at the time was talking to the care team about his goals for the day. The physician held up a finger silencing the patient, and placed a stethoscope to the patient's neck. The physician listened carefully for a moment, put down the stethoscope, told the patient he was doing very well, and left the room. The team, including the patient and family members, looked at one another in stunned silence. Gradually, the conversation resumed, but the spell had been broken.

During another observation a similar event happened. The collaborative team was functioning well, conversing with a patient recovering from heart surgery. A research team member with special training in teamwork observations noted a remarkably high level of team interaction in his research notes.

As this was happening, the patient's private physician came into the room. He looked quickly at the rounds team, then raised his hand in a dismissive gesture. "You will have to leave now," he said. The conversation collapsed, and the team filed out of the room with their heads down as if they were ashamed.

In both of these stories the care team talked about the events immediately after they occurred and later during their team meetings. These situations are difficult for many reasons. They revealed the differences in perspectives that exist, and they exposed the extent of power asymmetries that remain a reality in most care environments, even very advanced ones.

There are no easy answers presently, except to emphasize that when paradigms shift, there will be inevitable moments that are uncomfortable, and that the social landscape of health care is evolving and changing, slowly but steadily, for the better.

It may be helpful for your team to consider that this is still a pioneering time in health care, with all that pioneers must experience and endure, and that collaborative care is a pioneering innovation with inherent risks and difficulties.

Patience and respect

Our experience is that a growing number of physicians and organizational leaders are finding collaborative care exciting and worth changing expectations and work patterns to achieve.

Our recommendation is to look for the willing and work primarily with them. It is not usually productive or effective to try to challenge people in a confrontational way. The maxim of Gandhi to, "Be the change you wish to see in the world" applies to collaborative care. Invite people, yet resist the temptation to try to convert the unconverted. Simply show them a better way.

Find those who are interested and willing, and go forward with them. Remember that this takes time and patience.

Collaborative care is built best through respectful invitations. Don't give up, because people WILL change. The path to success is almost always through patience and learning over time.

Also, remember that the social risks of change are high for many people. If you are naturally visionary, these risks may not be so apparent to you. But for many people in the care environment, there is an ongoing social calculation about participating in the collaborative care initiative. When collaborative care is felt to be socially safe, people will embrace it. Like everything else, this shift happens over time as a relational accomplishment.

Summary of things your team can do to connect with the larger organization

Relationships between the local care environment and the larger organization can be given thoughtful attention, and effective connections can be intentionally and proactively developed.

- You can take time to discuss who will notice and who will be affected by the changes your team is making, and seek to develop relationships with those areas and people.
- You can look for synergies between what your team is accomplishing and initiatives throughout the organization, then align your efforts in mutually supportive ways.
- You can seek invitations to existing forums hosted by other parts of the organization to talk about why and what you are doing, and learn from others about their interests.
- You can intentionally establish relationships before making requests of other areas, and take into consideration your understanding of their goals and work flows.
- You can invite a transparent response from other parts of the organization about the impact that your work is having, and look for ways to manage their perceptions proactively.

- You can look for opportunities to represent your organization, and demonstrate to others how the success of your care environment supports organizational goals in innovative ways.
- You can invite organizational leaders to attend and experience collaborative rounds and weekly team meetings to further their understanding of collaborative care.
- You can open your doors to anyone who wants to participate in and learn about what you are doing on your unit, positioning yourselves as co-learners.
- You can identify strengths that have organizational currency – quality, efficiency, patient safety, and patient satisfaction – and position your work using these as leading indicators.
- If conflicts arise, draw attention to commonalities rather than differences, and remember that change takes time and has cycles of loss as well as progress. Be patient and respectful.

Simulation and Interprofessional Education

One of the most delightful experiences that a researcher or practitioner interested in collaborative care can have is teaching and modeling collaborative care with students from different health professions. In less than half a day of guided experience, working and reflecting together across professions in care scenarios with patients and family members, interprofessional student teams are able to reach remarkable levels of awareness and capability.

The experiences of teaching and participating in these sessions reinforce that collaborative care is natural for people and easily achieved from an ordinary human perspective. Any barriers to its adoption in established clinical environments arise mostly from years of prior training and deeply ingrained culture. If health care only had students, most of this book would not be needed.

In traditional health care, methods of education and practice are aligned in ways that support traditional care. When health professions students train separately from one another, the same processes of social construction that build collaborative care in collaborative environments will also build traditional care when students are isolated by role during their formative interactions.

We have found that introducing students to collaborative care is eye-opening for established professionals in an emerging collaborative care environment. The students take it up naturally. A story that illustrates this is from a care team that was trying to intentionally talk with patients and families on rounds using the pronoun “you,” rather than reporting about the patient as “he” or “she” in a traditional way. It was immediately clear to the care team that students and new graduates could do this effortlessly, while more experienced care team members often struggled to do this and frequently lapsed back into a familiar mode of reporting.

Formative and generative

Interprofessional education provides a new foundation of experiences, and generates different kinds of formative interactions and conversations for students and teachers alike. In a similar and additive way, health care simulation is remarkably effective as a pathway for exploring new ways of working while minimizing risk, both for patients and health care professionals.

It is increasingly clear that how people work together in actual care environments and how health professions students are educated should be considered together as an inseparable whole. An entire book could be written about interprofessional education and simulation. This is not that book, however the synergies and connections between interprofessional education, simulation, and collaborative care are important to consider.

Something very beautiful

Before reflecting about the nuances of these topics, let's take a moment to appreciate what becomes possible when health professions students train together. These experiences can be life-changing for everyone involved.

In just a morning or afternoon together, stereotypes, preconceptions, fears, and worries about working with other health professions, patients and families, can disappear. These feelings are replaced by new knowledge about others' roles and abilities, new awareness of shared purposes, and growing mutual respect.

The photograph below shows a simulation learning activity involving an interprofessional team of medical students, nursing students, pharmacy students, and respiratory therapy students together with an interactive patient manikin and family members.

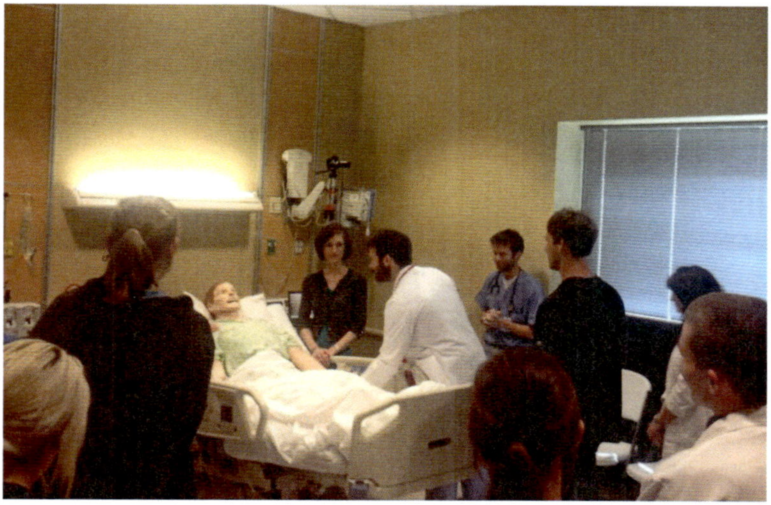

Figure: Collaborative care simulation with interprofessional student teams

The simulation sessions were held in an intensive care unit. Actors at the bedside played the roles of the patient's family members. The person providing the voice of the patient manikin could listen and speak as the patient with everyone in the room.

The simulations allowed the students to try out various ways of working together, followed by debriefings in which students were able to learn from each other about their thoughts and experiences. As is always the case, students from every profession were surprised and reassured to learn that students from other professions were just as nervous and uncertain as they were. In successive scenarios the students explored many ways of working together interprofessionally and of actively engaging the patient and family members in care and decision making.

Throughout the day, the interprofessional faculty of three nurses, a physician, a paramedic, and two faculty members who are not health care professionals modeled respectful interactions and encouraged the students to reflect about their experiences together. The actors playing the patient and family members participated in the debriefings and talked with the students about how they felt and what they experienced during the scenarios.

The students, faculty, and the care team members in the care environment where the simulations were held were all changed in lasting ways by participating in these experiences. There is something very powerful about watching others exploring these kinds of interactions. Simulation allows people to see things they might not recognize when they in the middle of actual care. The experiences and reflections linger long after the event is over.

The importance of patient voice and family presence

In your simulation activities in support of collaborative care, we encourage you to intentionally include patient voice and the presence of family members in all of your scenarios, and to always include discussions about active patient and family engagement in your scenario planning and debriefings.

We have observed that there can be a tendency, even among people very dedicated to patient and family engagement, to focus in simulation on medical and technical details of care. This often extends to technical details of teamwork among health professionals, which often are taught as competencies and behaviors that can be taught and tested in simulation settings.

It takes thoughtful attention on everyone's part to actively include a focus on patient and family engagement in the planning and design of every scenario, and to include discussions about patient and family engagement during every debriefing.

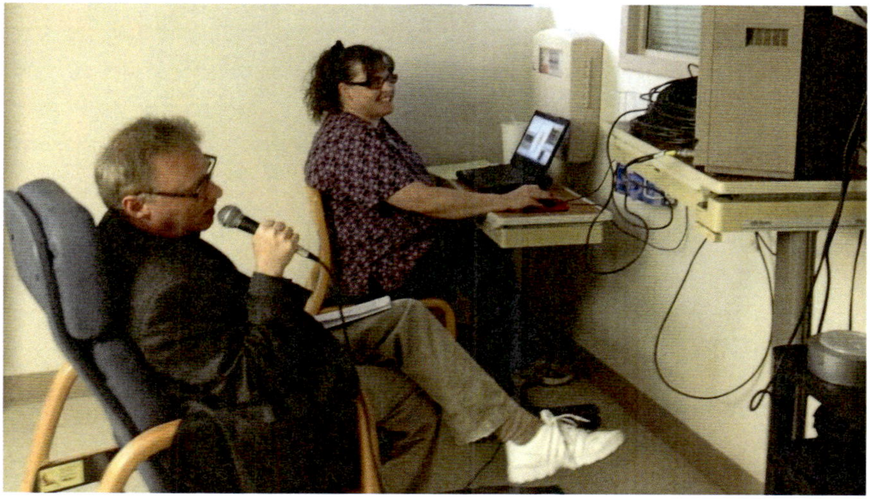

Figure: Voice of the patient from the simulation control room

We prefer to use scenarios where conversations and physiologic events change in response to learner actions as these unfold in real time. We utilize a pattern whenever possible of beginning each scenario with a stable first setting, during which the professional care team members can meet the patient and family members in a relaxed manner. We remind the team members participating in the scenario to treat the simulation environment as an actual clinical space, and reinforce this by encouraging actions including washing hands, introducing themselves to the patient and family, and asking permission to ask questions and examine the patient.

We start the action of the scenario before the professional care team members enter the room, encouraging the patient, family members and bedside nurse to immerse comfortably in their characters as people, talking and interacting as they would if they were actually in the hospital.

We then bring in the team members that will be responding in the scenario, inviting them to meet the patient and family and encouraging everyone to introduce themselves and take a few minutes to interact by having a conversation with the patient as a person. We also use this time to make clear what is real and what is not in terms of physical exam, monitors, location of supplies, and so forth.

After several more minutes of comfortable interaction, we have the professional care team members leave the room, reset the action, and the designed scenario begins.

We have found that attention to these details and the small investment of time required for doing this produce tremendous benefits. The interactions take on a human quality and richness that helps everyone involved.

Part of the power of the simulation experience is the human connections that develop among everyone present when conducted in these ways.

Simulation and the growth of collaborative capabilities

When we first began studying collaborative care, we thought it would be possible to train people in certain things like collaborative rounds, have people practice these things in ways including simulation, then send people out into the world expecting to see better outcomes wherever people trained in these ways were able to work together. It didn't work out quite like that. That story is partly right, but it misses something very important.

As we first began this work, we did not recognize the importance of the way that the collaborative care environment develops over time. Another way of saying this is that we were able to see teams working together, but we were not able to see and appreciate the development of how they got that way.

Because we were not able, at first, to visualize the development of the care environment and how that happens through ongoing interactions and conversations of the care team, we did not fully appreciate that collaborative care is more than the sum of trainable individual teamwork behaviors. It is entirely possible to train people in individual teamwork skills, have team members participate in an interprofessional multidisciplinary rounds process, and fall far short of the expectations of reliability and resilience that collaborative care promises.

What is missing is the development of contextual resources that arise through cumulative experiences and ongoing reflective conversations of a care team that is able to work and learn together over time. Individual teamwork skills are only the beginning of that process of growth and development, and as our research suggests, are perhaps not the most important factor.

As our understanding of collaborative care has deepened, our attention has shifted beyond the individual learner to the development of specific teams in their local environments, as a whole. This is quite a significant distinction, since a lot of simulation training and even competencies for interprofessional education often focus on capabilities of the individual learner.

Interprofessional education experiences and simulation-based teamwork experiences are helpful for developing and sustaining collaborative care, no matter how they are done. But it is easy to focus on individual teamwork behaviors and miss the importance of the growth of collaborative capabilities over time through educational experiences and reflective conversations of a particular care team. To be truly effective for developing reliability and resilience, interprofessional education and simulation need to be conducted for specific teams, as well as for individual learners.

This distinction between teamwork training that focuses on individual teamwork behaviors, and teamwork training that truly focuses on teams, needs to be more fully explored in research and enacted in recommended practices of health care simulation. The short version, though, is that anything your team does together, especially interprofessional education and simulation, will help sustain your collaborative care environment.

We have included interprofessional education and simulation in this section about sustaining collaborative care rather than in an earlier section about deepening collaborative care, because sustaining collaborative care involves and requires fundamental shifts of thought and practice. In the same way that organizational structures and operational models need to be different in order to sustain collaborative care, educational models and even research methods need to be different as well.

Becoming a Model for Others

One of the most helpful things your team can do to sustain collaborative care is to become a model for others. Becoming a model for others can go hand-in-hand with your own continuous learning. For example, asking your team how you are collectively doing with "inviting and welcoming" is a natural moment to actually invite and welcome others into your work environment.

There is power in a pattern of interaction that invites, welcomes, opens to vulnerable observation, listens to new voices, and notices the response of others. Others will see things you might not. Modeling and sharing your experiences becomes an opportunity to see through another's eyes. Aliveness can be served by creating opportunities to describe for others what you are doing together as a team, and what you are most proud of.

Invite your team to create a presentation that highlights your contextual resources as these grow and develop. Talk about your GLITCH process and what you have learned. Tell about how gathering your own data has helped. Talking with others will build appreciation for why your work is meaningful. Sometimes teams don't realize the significance of their work until they do this. Remember to talk about what surprised you. Surprises are a reminder that our assumptions are just that, assumptions.

Visitors and presentations are opportunities to tell stories about when being alert, patient, and responsive as a team paid off, or how engaging the patient and family made an important difference. Use real, concrete stories about your experiences. Engaging others acknowledges the relational aspect of everything we do. Becoming a model means engaging others in the ongoing process of co-creating your collaborative care environment.

PART SEVEN

SOCIAL FIELD MODEL

- Social Fields
- Contextual Resources
- Social Construction
- Relational Infrastructure
- Social Field Model of Collaborative Care

Social Fields

To help understand and implement collaborative care, we found it useful to develop a concept we call social fields.

Every human being has experienced social fields. We have all been present when a hush falls over an audience at a special moment. We have been part of a crowd that leaps to its feet cheering in unison. We have experienced the transcendence of being part of a group of people united by singing, or have been on a team able to reach exceptional levels of performance. We know immediately when certain people have a special closeness – we sense it in the way they interact.

These are manifestations of social fields.

The concept of social fields is a way of visualizing and talking about human connections that can grow, and the richness of experience that is available, in a well-developed collaborative environment, including the accumulated knowledge, wisdom, humor, and patterns of interaction that arise and develop among a team that works and learns together over time.

Before we started to think in terms of social fields, we were searching for familiar experiences from ordinary life that could help Illustrate the kind of connections we were trying to describe. One day the experience of a "knowing smile" occurred to us.

A Knowing Smile

We immediately recognized that a "knowing smile" could help communicate what we were trying to express about how great teams work. To understand social fields in collaborative care, it is helpful to think about knowing smiles.

A knowing smile is a look between people that signifies much more than is obvious. With a quick glance, a twinkle of an eye, a tilt of the head or some other meaningful expression – in those simple gestures – an entire past history of information, memory, emotions, and shared experiences can flow between people, often without a word being spoken. As human beings we have all experienced knowing smiles and have watched them brighten the space between others.

It is interesting to reflect about what makes knowing smiles possible, and what they accomplish. It is also interesting to reflect about how hard it would be to communicate everything carried in a knowing smile if knowing smiles did not exist.

Let's think first about what must happen before people can share a knowing smile.

It is certainly possible for people to share a smile who have never met one another. Even when meeting for the first time, people can make sense of a smile. Most of the time a smile means happiness, friendliness, and a certain degree of openness. We know this from a lifetime of learning as we have interacted with others. So, there is a certain baseline of shared experience that lets us share a smile, just from being human.

But the kind of knowing smile we are talking about here carries even more than this. Before a knowing smile is possible, people must have some shared experience together, enough that a special kind of insight and meaning becomes woven into their interactions and can be communicated, acknowledged and affirmed by the simple gesture of a smile. In other words, a knowing smile has a history.

People who share knowing smiles must know one another. The memories and connections that flow between people in a knowing smile have been built over time through shared experiences together. In the context of this shared history, many things become possible that would not be possible otherwise.

In the same way that a knowing smile becomes possible, the special capabilities of collaborative care develop through shared experiences as a care team works and learns together. The capabilities of the team grow and become available to the team in its daily interactions, making the work of the team easier and giving it special meaning.

A social field can be thought of as a living collective intelligence that grows over time among members of a team who are able to work together regularly. The experiences and connections that develop in a care environment become familiar and available to the people who create them together.

A team with a well-developed social field can draw upon these connections and shared history in its work together. Like a knowing smile, many things become possible in a well-developed social field that would not be possible otherwise, and almost effortlessly so.

Social fields develop over time if conditions are right

We have found it helpful to reflect about the growth of a social field among a group of people over time.

At first, as people are just starting to work together and getting to know one another, their social field is not very well developed. As people are able to work together consistently and come to know one another better, a reservoir of shared history develops and it becomes easier to work together. People learn what to expect by doing things together, and carry with them what they have learned. Their social field is developing.

The figure below illustrates this growth of a social field from early "transactional" interactions to a richly developed social field:

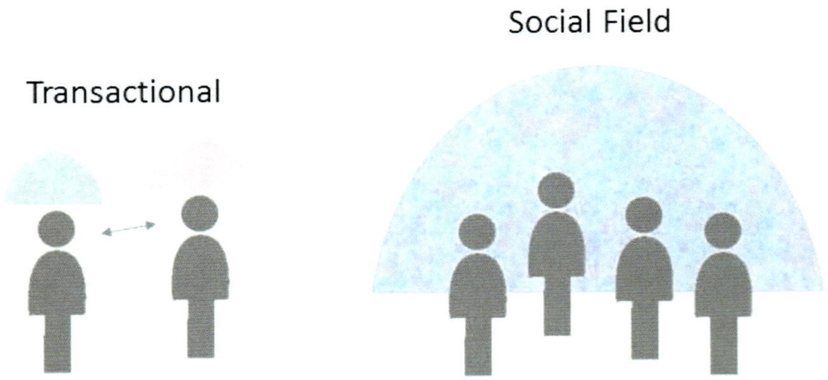

Figure: Before and after the development of a social field

The people represented on the right side of the figure have worked together before, know one another, and have an accumulated history of shared experiences, collective knowledge, and mutual insights from their previous interactions together. This accumulated knowledge of what to expect and do is represented by the multicolored space that surrounds them – their social field.

In contrast, the people represented on the left side of the figure do not have a well-developed social field. They have individual professional role knowledge and expertise represented by the colored spaces over each person. However, individual expertise is all they are able to contribute. They haven't worked together as a true team before. They do not have prior shared experiences they can draw from in their work together. Their interactions must be transactionally coordinated because they haven't developed shared collective knowledge yet.

Working without a social field requires a lot of effort. The only way to make sure things are clear between people is to precisely specify everything. It can be exhausting to work like that. Without a social field, tomorrow is just as hard as today, because very little is carried forward. In fact, tomorrow can become very discouraging, because most of what was said yesterday has to be said all over again, every time. A lot of health care is like that.

Our research suggests that many dimensions of the "goodness" of exceptional care teams – including reliability and resilience as well as human dimensions of compassion and caring – depend a lot on the development of rich social fields. The social field of a care team is made up of experiences and patterns of interaction that the team can draw upon based on their shared history together – resources for connecting, coordinating, learning, making decisions, managing differences – and many other things they need to do as a team that they have "made" together in prior interactions. A care team in a well-developed social field can do much of this without words, often without conscious thought.

"Best days"

Another way to think about social fields is to reflect about your "best days" at work. One of the things we enjoy in our research is asking people about their best days. People usually smile, nod, then tell us about what happens on their best days.

Almost always, people mention two things about their best days. The first thing is how happy they are on their best days. Work feels more meaningful on those days. Another thing people talk about is the people they enjoy working with. When people reflect about their best days, they usually describe being part of a trusted group of people who work especially well together. One person said, "When I am working with these people, I just know it is going to be a great day. I trust them and they trust me. We are seamless and things just really flow. Everything is easier."

Try asking yourself or a friend about "best days." We think you will quickly see what we mean. As a research team, we smile a knowing smile when people talk about their best days, because we know that they are describing a really great social field.

Tacit knowledge at a team level

To take this concept of social fields farther, it is helpful to consider the difference between explicit knowledge and tacit knowledge. Explicit knowledge is knowledge that can be written down. Tacit knowledge, which is a different kind of knowledge, is an ability to get things done. Tacit knowledge is learned from experience. Knowing what to do is not the same as being able to do it. Researchers who study expertise and mastery point to rich tacit knowledge as the thing that experts have that novices don't.

There is a lot of interest in society about tacit knowledge and what it takes to achieve mastery of a professional or skill. The literature about deliberate practice is part of this conversation. It is often said that it takes 10,000 hours of deliberate practice to achieve mastery of a highly developed skill like playing the violin.

Even at a more basic level of ordinary life experience, tacit knowledge is very important. Think about your first day in a new work environment when you didn't even know where to find supplies. Times like that are frustrating and discouraging. Soon, you develop tacit knowledge and work becomes much easier.

Expertise depends on tacit knowledge. As we gain tacit knowledge, we can scan for patterns that fit our expectations of a situation and rapidly focus in on the things that matter most. We can sense when things are going well, and of equal importance, we can know when things are not going well, because we know from past experience what things should be like. With rich tacit knowledge we can do ordinary work effortlessly, almost without conscious thought, saving our explicit attention for the things that are unique and require special focus.

Now, let's transition from individual tacit knowledge to tacit knowledge at the level of the team as a whole. Individual tacit knowledge is important, but that is already a given in health care. What we are concerned with for reliability and resilience is tacit knowledge at a team level. Both levels matter, but what matters most for exceptional teamwork is how tacit knowledge arises for an entire team collectively, beyond the tacit knowledge of each individual team member.

Just like an individual person, a team has to do things together and learn from experience for tacit knowledge to develop. If a team is able to work together on a regular basis in a supportive environment, and, especially, if people have time to reflect together about what they are doing, they will learn and get really good at what they do. However, if a team doesn't work together consistently, tacit knowledge can't develop very well.

Social field as rich tacit context

The concept of social fields is useful for understanding how rich tacit knowledge develops for a team. The tacit knowledge of a team is carried and expressed in its social field. A social field is a context rich with tacit knowledge of many kinds. People in well-developed social fields rely on familiar patterns of interaction to know what to expect and how to make sense of their experiences. People understand how to respond in any particular circumstance – know what ought to be done – based on what they have seen and experienced before in similar situations.

Being in a rich tacit environment makes doing routine things easy, and enhances the ability of the team to do critical things that require special consideration and special focus. When a team has built up a lot of tacit knowledge together, routine things take almost no effort. Tacit knowledge clears away the routine forest, allowing each important special tree to be clearly seen.

Working together as a team consistently over time is essential for team-level tacit knowledge to develop. Adding regular opportunities for a team to meet and reflect together as a normal part of their work together will accelerate how quickly team-level tacit knowledge in a social field develops. Once developed, the tacit knowledge in a social field is quite powerful. Our experience suggests that people respond to social fields and socialize into them without a great deal of thought or effort simply by being present and participating in them. The tacit knowledge carried in the social field becomes "the way we do things around here."

Once a social field is established, life within the social field becomes easier for people. Ideas can be communicated with reference to past experience more fluently, and often this can even happen without conscious attention. People know what to expect and do with each other. Team members, patients and family members are able to function together in exceptional ways.

All kinds of human knowledge and emotions

Social fields can carry all kinds of knowledge and emotions, not just knowledge about how to do things. The social fields that we have experienced in well-developed collaborative care are remarkably rich with every dimension of human wisdom and insight, including empathy and humor. As we have mentioned earlier, laughter is a hallmark of collaborative care.

When a care team has developed a strong collaborative social field, people feel and respond to it. It is a sensibility that guides people, a felt sense of connection with known patterns.

The social field of a highly evolved collaborative team can be thought of as a living collective intelligence, or even as a life force. In our research, patients and family members experience and talk about relating with the collaborative care team as they might describe a special relationship with an individual person.

Local and constantly changing

This understanding of social fields, as carrying rich tacit knowledge that becomes "the way we do things around here," is an exciting way of understanding culture and the localness of culture that is seen in health care. Consider, for example, the notable differences in safety attitudes that have been shown between different units in the same hospital. Rather than viewing culture as a fixed and static property of the organization as a whole, it is interesting to visualize social fields as being constantly made and remade by the ongoing interactions and conversations of people working together in a particular local care environment.

From a social field perspective, what is called culture is locally made and constantly in motion. The pathway for changing culture is by modifying the interactions and conversations in the care environment that continuously form and re-form the local social field. This can be accomplished by changing preconditions that shape how these interactions and conversations occur.

To summarize, we believe that highly reliable and resilient collaborative care teams that are able to actively engage patients and family members are functioning in highly developed social fields, rich with contextual resources that enable them to take exceptional care of patients and each other. *The Field Guide to Collaborative Care* has been written to help care teams intentionally develop and bring to life these vibrant, resource-rich social fields in their own care environments.

Contextual Resources

The capabilities that arise and enable collaborative care are developed through team-level interactions and conversations. We chose the name "Contextual Resources" for these capabilities because they are resources that become available to the team over time in the context of a social field with its own local history.

We believe that the extent and nature of contextual resources in social fields is what distinguishes exceptional collaborative care teams. Contextual resources are experienced by patients, families and care team members in many ways, including ease of working together, enhanced individual and collective knowledge, and as collective expressions of kindness, empathy, wisdom and humor.

Contextual resources arise and develop locally through ongoing cycles of action and reflection. Creating contextual resources is an ongoing process of mutual shaping and reshaping what makes sense and has meaning for people in a particular care context. The effects and benefits are not just for the people initially involved, but for anyone who is able to participate in the conversations and reflections as these propagate, enabling and reshaping the care environment.

Eight contextual resources which we believe are important for resilience and reliability are presented on the following pages, using narrative descriptions from our interviews and observations.

Resource 1: Knowing what to Expect and Do

Description: "We have a collective intelligence as a team. From our experience working together, we have developed a deep knowledge of the situations we usually encounter and what is needed in those situations. We can see a bigger picture and know how to integrate with that. We have learned how our team will respond, and how to coordinate with each other. We know when things are normal, when things are abnormal in ways we have experienced before, and when things are abnormal in ways we have never experienced before. We know what to do in each of those situations. This understanding extends beyond what to expect and do medically, to other dimensions of our interactions together, including empathy and caring. If you were to watch us work, you see a fluid kind of leadership. All of us have the ability to contribute and lead, depending on what we are doing at the time."

Resource 2: Alertness/Responsiveness/Patience

Description: "Our team is alert and responsive and patient in ways that let us work really well together. We have many things that we could be doing that compete for our attention, and there is a lot of work to get done. Yet when we need to respond as a team to something – for example, when we need to go into action quickly, or slow down to really figure something out, or listen carefully to a concern of a patient or family member, we are really good at doing that together. We can be in one routine one minute, then shift on the spot to an entirely different mode of interaction when that becomes necessary. We are alert and responsive and patient when something changes and we need to go fast, and also when we need to go slow or change course. We do things in real time. Nobody comes into any situation thinking they know what to do or will be told. We figure things out together."

Resource 3: Ability to Invite and Welcome

Description: "One of the notable things about our team is our ability to invite and welcome. There are certain things we do – for example, how we introduce ourselves on rounds and ask patients about their personal interests – that help us welcome new people into our routines. We have figured out how to have a spirit of Inclusion. People who are new to our team, and patients and families, too, usually feel like they belong as part of our team right away. There is an expectation here that everyone has something to contribute, even the newest or quietest voice. We seek those out. And we are comfortable that people will have differing perspectives. Most of the time we are able to talk openly and comfortably about our differences. We see these as sources of insight. We are also able to talk openly about hard things like mistakes, or death. We have become comfortable with that. One person said, "I saw you treating other people well, and me too, and then I believed it." There is a sense of openness and transparency and curiosity about new people and new ideas that is comfortable and respectful. We have an interest in knowing about each other and seeing the good in each other that is welcoming and nonjudgmental."

Resource 4: Commitment to Learning and Change

Description: "There is an excitement here about learning. We are learning together all the time as an interprofessional team, including patients and families. We truly get it that we are a team, and that our outcomes are something we achieve together. We intentionally monitor how we are doing, and are always looking for ways to do even better. We change things together. We have a strong drive to excel, combined with a spirit and confidence to "just try it and see what emerges." It is part of us. Our different viewpoints mesh together and allow us to generate new ideas. That is one of our greatest strengths. We have a shared commitment to that. The shift from a nay-saying culture to a yes-saying culture is something we worked hard to make happen. You can feel it here."

Resource 5: Engagement with Patients and Families

Description: "It is interesting how we relate with patients and families here. Our patients are not just patients to us. We become part of each other in a very interesting way. One family member tried to describe what that was like. She said, "There is this 'crossing over'." She meant that their needs become our needs, and our needs become their needs. It is equal. This goes beyond involving patients and family members in medical decisions. It is about more than that. At first that surprised us, but not anymore. We are attentive to their medical care, of course. But what we really focus on is what matters as people. The real work is about meaning. The sister of one of our patients was getting married. It mattered to him to be there, more than anything else. We got him there."

Resource 6: A Web of Monitoring

Description: "Part of why our outcomes are so good is that everyone here is on the same page and devoting attention to things together. If something isn't going like we expected it should, we are able to recognize that right away. Someone will see something, even if it is not in their area of expertise, and everyone feels comfortable bringing things to the attention of others. Because we know what is supposed to happen, and are connected and comfortable with one another, when something isn't going right we are able to see that very early and respond right away to get things back on track. There is also an attitude here of not being complacent. We are always asking ourselves, "What are we missing here? Is there anything else that might be happening? How are we being led down the path of not seeing something?" The holes in our web are very small. We catch things."

Resource 7: Emergence

Description: "One of the most interesting things here is how often new ideas and unexpected insights emerge in the course of our interactions and conversations with one another. Many of these new ideas weren't in the mind of anyone before we began. We experience this on rounds during our assessment process and in our planning and decision making, and we also see it in other meetings together. Because we are all together and able to communicate so well and comfortably, our interactions are very generative. One person's idea triggers another person's new idea, and before you know it, as a collective team we are seeing things completely differently with new insights we would never have had before. We have learned to expect that will happen. We count on it."

Resource 8: Aliveness

Description: "You can feel the aliveness here when you get off the elevator. One thing that makes this a great place is the opportunities here for each person to make contributions, and how much you are respected and appreciated for that. People recognize when you give something of yourself, and everyone makes sure you know it matters. It takes time and effort to do that, and we make time. Being able to contribute that way makes you feel really good. It restores you as a person. The first feeling when something happens is usually appreciation, not criticism or frustration. We laugh a lot together. One person said, "A key test is the effect on the human spirit. Do the things we are doing together support or oppress the human spirit?" That is true. That is how we care for patients and families, and for each other. Our attention to the human spirit underlies all of our good results."

Social Construction

It is interesting to study the "what" of exceptional health care, such as descriptions of exceptional teamwork. Yet, these descriptions are useful only if they can be brought to life with the "how" of collaborative care – practical methods for successfully implementing and sustaining collaborative care.

In our work and research, our understanding about how collaborative care can be successfully implemented has been greatly influenced by a field of scholarship known as Social Construction. The focus of social construction is on what people collectively do and talk about together, and what these interactions and conversations make, or socially construct.

Social construction assumes that understandings and meaning are developed in relationship with others, and that actions flow from these. From a social construction perspective, collaborative care doesn't happen from an intent or mandate to be collaborative, or from training. Rather, collaborative care is socially constructed as care team members, patients, and family members do things together, reflect, and talk together. Social construction emphasizes that what makes sense and what matters to people, and, therefore, what people do that flows from those beliefs and meaning, are explored and worked out – made socially – through ongoing experiences and reflective conversations with each other.

The insight of social construction regarding the "how" of collaborative care is that collaborative care flows from interactions and conversations in the care environment, and is shaped by preconditions in the environment that influence how the interactions and conversations happen and are experienced.

Interventions to create or strengthen collaborative care work best when they set the stage for new interactions and conversations of the care team. The goal is establishing optimum preconditions that will foster and support the kinds of interactions and conversations that are likely to lead to the emergence of collaborative care. This is different than focusing on collaborative practices themselves, or on individual behaviors.

Theories of social construction shift attention from desired individual behaviors and related concepts of motivation, incentives, and accountability, to the interactions and contexts that surround and guide individual behaviors – what the care environment is like, what people do together because of that, and what their actions and conversations create and make possible.

To make the idea of social construction more concrete, imagine a progression of events in a care environment as a nurse and a physician see a patient together; and, later, as the nurse and doctor talk about what happened with others. Imagine this begins as a doctor is especially kind to a patient and listens with respect and attention to the thoughts and suggestions of a nurse. After the doctor leaves, the nurse sits down with a colleague.

"You know, that doctor is really nice," the nurse says. "She listened to me and asked what I thought." Her colleague responds, "That happened to me, too." Another nurse adds, "Yes, me too. The patient said the doctor really seemed to care about her, and about what we think." After this the nurses go on with their work.

In these conversations the nurses are making sense and meaning out of what just happened. As they do so, they are constructing a belief that the doctor is great. They will carry this belief, and their feelings, with them after the conversation is over. The next time these nurses and that doctor work together, the nurses will bring these conversations and feelings with them. They will have a growing expectation that the doctor will listen and care. Responding to those expectations, the doctor may find it is especially nice to work with those nurses. She may tell someone, "You know, those nurses are really great to work with." The patients will notice, too, and add their comments. And so on. A virtuous cycle has started, making things better for everyone.

The doctor, nurses, and patients in these interactions and conversations will be influenced by their evolving mutual good expectations. What people experience and do is connected to what they have experienced and talked about before. Over time, a set of mutual expectations is continuously formed and re-formed, constructed and reconstructed among people, from their ongoing interactions and conversations. Perhaps a comment is made about a kindness shown. People will take note of that in their next interactions. These interactions will shape the care on that unit.

The example above emphasizes the growth of feelings, which are important in collaborative care. In addition to feelings, the same potential for growth and learning is also true for other kinds of human knowledge, and for the collective abilities of the care team to do things together – for example, monitoring the condition of a patient and responding if there is a problem or concern. The point is that all of these – emotions and perceptions of people in the care environment together with team-level capabilities to perceive and act – are built and develop over time as the team works and learns together. We believe that the special capabilities of exceptional teams, such as reliability and resilience, arise and develop this way.

It is important to recognize that this kind of learning can be intentionally influenced by many things. If people work together once but never again, the lessons learned don't have a way of accumulating and impacting care. However, if people are able to work consistently together, and if they have opportunities to talk and reflect together, it is likely they will progressively gain new insights about one another that can make working together easier.

By restructuring the care environment to provide for consistency of interactions and opportunities for the team reflection to reflect and talk together, these team-level capabilities can be intentionally created and strengthened. Social construction helps make clear that linkages exist between what people do together and how their next interactions will be shaped because of that. Social construction helps explain how this happens, and how all of these things are connected in useful ways. Social construction emphasizes that every interaction among the care team matters. This is true not only for what the care team does as it cares for patients together, but also for the interactions and conversations among care team members as they reflect together about what they are experiencing and doing.

From a social construction perspective, reflective conversations are an essential part of how people make sense and find meaning in what they are experiencing. What makes sense and has meaning is always evolving. What people do together, and what is being made by these interactions and conversations, always bring the potential of new possibilities.

The importance of reflective conversations

In our research we found that social construction was the magic key we were searching for that unlocked our understanding of how collaborative care is created. When we began to view collaborative care through a social construction lens, our focus shifted from the actions of the care team during care, to the interactions and reflective conversations that we could now understand were shaping and influencing the observable actions.

In time, we began to recognize that the "place to put the wrench" to transform a care environment is the reflective conversations of the care team, patients, and family members. We began to see that in most traditional care environments there are few opportunities for care team members, patients, and family members to reflect together about their interactions. Instead, people in these environments are just busy doing their work.

Reflective conversations were happening, of course, but almost always in isolated groups – nurses with other nurses, doctors with other doctors, patients and family members talking together among themselves during the course of their work day.

Using a social construction lens, we began to see that in most care environments there is a missing infrastructure for collaborative reflection at a team level. Most teams have no opportunity for meeting and talking in a mode of reflection, except in the moment-by-moment work of direct patient care when reflective conversations of the entire team are almost impossible.

We began to recognize that reflective conversations in regular team meetings were the place to begin to successfully implement collaborative care.

Relational Infrastructure

As we began to recognize the importance of having opportunities for reflective conversations at a team level, we began to think of these as an infrastructure in the work environment, usually absent, that was needed for collaborative care to grow and develop.

To communicate what we were seeing, we developed a term for the infrastructure necessary for collaborative care to develop. We chose the term "Relational Infrastructure."

We define relational infrastructure as anything in the care environment that allows people to interact and reflect together, "setting the stage" for collaborative care to emerge.

The concept of relational infrastructure provides a way of explaining why high reliability collaborative care arises in some clinical environments but not in others. It also provides insights about how care environments can be intentionally restructured to make collaborative care more likely to emerge. Relational infrastructure for collaborative care is anything in the care environment that provides opportunities for people to reflect and converse together across professions, ideally with active participation by patients and family members. For example, having weekly reflective team meetings is an example of relational infrastructure. Making daily collaborative rounds with patients and families is another example.

Closely connected with relational infrastructure are organizational practices that provide for stable and consistent team interactions; leadership that provides for respectful, open communication and creates psychological safety; and processes that support learning and system improvement at local team level. These infuse an aliveness of spirit that brings people together and catalyzes the development of collaborative working relationships among professional team members, patients and families. Certain environments have more of these elements than others. These environments have a "natural" infrastructure for exceptional teamwork. An example discussed before might be a closely staffed ICU where people work together regularly and consistently, and leaders by nature are open and engaging.

Collaborative care is easier to implement on a unit that has natural relational infrastructure, such as the closely staffed ICU, and much more difficult to implement on another unit with multiple services and different conflicting schedules, where a social field is basically prevented from forming by the way the unit is organized.

The opposite example might be the med-surg unit we discussed before, where team members have no way to get to know one another well. The more we look at traditional care environments in our research, the more we recognize "structural holes" where relational infrastructure should exist but doesn't.

If relational infrastructure is carefully assessed and strengthened as part of initial efforts to implement collaborative care in the care environment, the efforts are much more likely to be successful. Relational infrastructure is the structural foundation upon which collaborative care is built.

Social Field Model of Collaborative Care

We hope that in these discussions you are beginning to see that concepts of *social fields, tacit knowledge, social construction, contextual resources, cycles of action-reflection learning, relational infrastructure, and collaborative leadership* can be brought together as a way of understanding how collaborative care works and how it can be intentionally implemented.

The *Social Field Model of Collaborative Care* is a theoretical and practical model for understanding and implementing collaborative care. It can also be used to inform research about collaborative care and for studying the emergence of reliability and resilience. The model has three layers, or views, of collaborative care, described in the following sections.

Layer One: What is collaborative care?

Layer One, below, illustrates the essential elements of collaborative care which are 1) active engagement of patients and families, 2) exceptional teamwork across the entire interprofessional team, and 3) active learning to achieve reliability and resilience. The figure also identifies foundational elements of the Social Field Model of Collaborative Care.

The most important of these – that a social field is the context for collaborative care – is shown at the top in words beneath a demarcating, curved line.

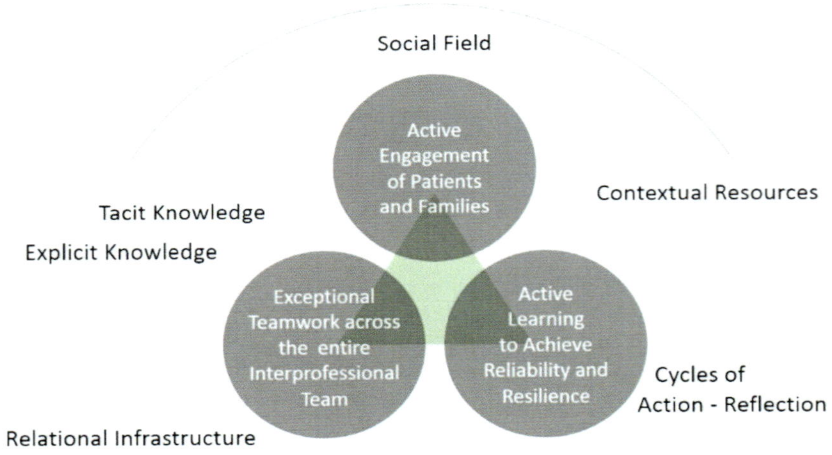

Layer One: Foundational elements
Social Field Model of Collaborative Care

The curved line emphasizes that collaborative care is local and historical, arising among a certain group of people in a particular care context over time. The capabilities of reliability and resilience emerge and develop in the social field as these are created by people interacting, talking, and learning together.

In the Layer One diagram, the words outside of the circles are important for understanding how collaborative care grows and develops. From the lower left these words are Relational Infrastructure, Explicit Knowledge, Tacit Knowledge, Social Field, Contextual Resources, and Cycles of Action-Reflection. These are the basic building blocks of the social field model.

Layer two: "How does it work?"

If you could walk into the second layer you would feel like you are entering a factory or a foundry. People are doing things together and making things together in the second layer.

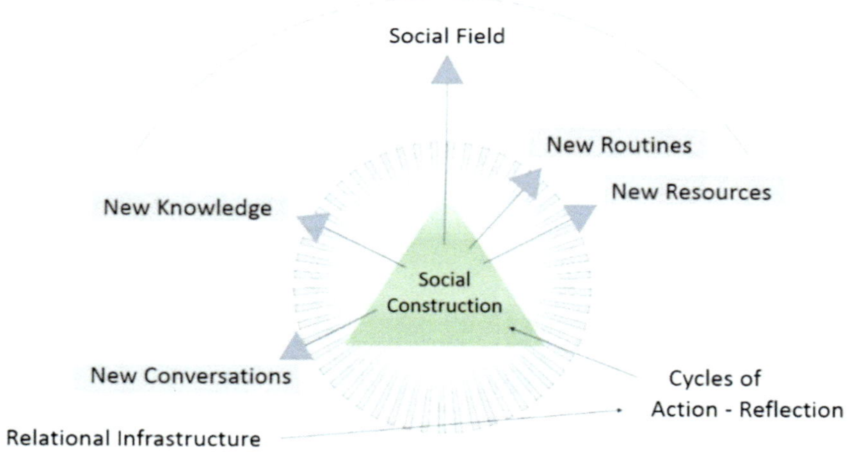

Layer Two: Antecedents and effects of social construction
Social Field Model of Collaborative Care

At the center of Layer Two is a green triangle called "social construction" that radiates throughout the social field. As we described in an earlier section, social construction focuses on how things are made – socially constructed – as people interact and converse together. The green triangle of social construction guides attention to the importance of people doing things together and making contextual resources together by their ongoing interactions and conversations.

A major point of Layer Two is how the interactions and conversations of the care team socially construct the special capabilities of collaborative care. This is illustrated by the arrows that radiate outward into the social field as people in the care environment interact and converse. As people interact, the social field grows and changes. New conversations become possible, new knowledge is created, new routines are established, and new contextual resources are generated

Layer Two shows that the interactions of the care team working and conversing with one another and with patients and families, and the preconditions that make these make possible, are the heart and soul of collaborative care. The figure also shows that the interactions and conversations of the care team are shaped by relational infrastructure, and action-reflection learning.

Through ongoing interactions and conversations of the care team, and all that becomes possible because of them, a collaborative social field progressively develops, and the capabilities that emerge and grow there increase and expand.

Collaborative care is implemented by intentionally connecting elements of relational infrastructure together so that a care team is able to participate in ongoing cycles of action and reflection. This means *action* together, such as daily collaborative rounds, and also *reflection* together, such as weekly team meetings where the team can make sense of what they are doing together and consider how things could be even better.

Social construction underlies everything that happens in collaborative care, and preconditions set the stage for social construction. Preconditions are the key leverage points. Put the wrench on the preconditions and you will change things.

Layer three: "Why does it work?"

Layer Three, illustrated in the figure below, is more theory-based. It builds upon concepts of social fields, contextual resources, relational infrastructure, social construction and action-reflection learning from the first two layers of the model, adding concepts of *sensemaking and meaning making* to the model.

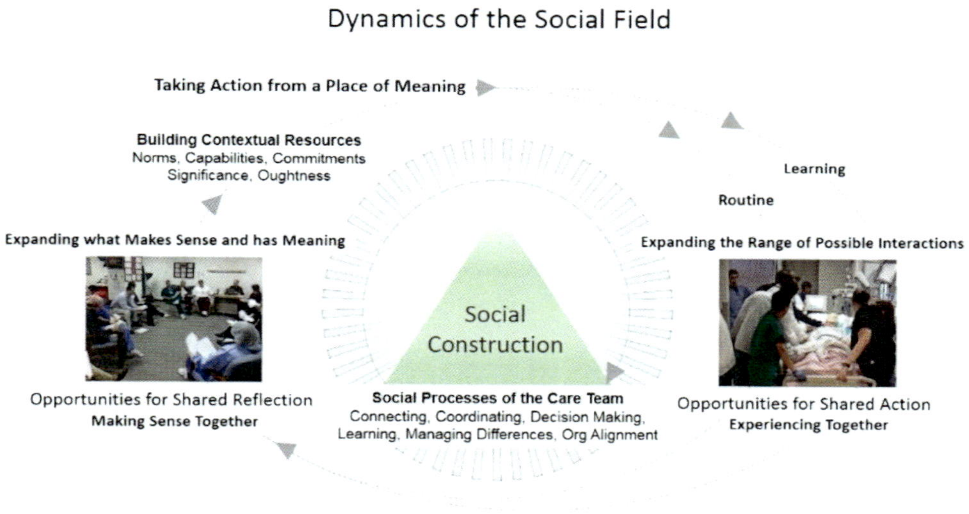

Layer Three: Reconstructing social processes of the care team
Social Field Model of Collaborative Care

This layer considers even more deeply why collaborative care works by focusing on the development of patterns of interaction of the care team – ways of *connecting, coordinating, making decisions, learning, managing differences, and aligning with the larger organization,* which are called social processes.

Social processes can occur in many ways. In collaborative care the social processes of the care team happen differently than in traditional practice. They are more welcoming, inviting, participatory, and affirming of the human spirit. Layer Three emphasizes the dynamics of the social processes of the care team, and how these social processes form and change over time.

The question for a researcher interested in implementing collaborative care is why the social processes of a care team happen as they do, and related to that, how social processes can develop and evolve in ways that generate collaboration and the contextual resources that enable high reliability and resilience.

Consider the diagram of Layer Three, which is an illustration of a dynamic process of continuous change and development. This view of collaborative care emphasizes that every social field is a continuously evolving and changing context. The inner loop of the field represents the usual routines of the care team. The outer loop represents a state of active learning.

The flows of Layer Three emphasize that a care team is always moving in generative loops of ongoing experiences and reflections that have consequences for what happens next. Ongoing flows of action and reflection create the social processes of the care team – ways of connecting, coordinating, and so forth, with social construction as the way these processes are made.

The flows also generate contextual resources – the norms, capabilities, commitments, felt significance, and oughtness of those ways of relating. Everything arises in, is shaped by, and influences the interactions and conversations of the care team. Everything is connected by what makes sense and has meaning in the social field – which also change with the ongoing flows.

Layer Three illustrates continuous dynamics that have no starting point or ending point. However, a good way to understand this layer is to enter into the illustration at the top of the flows, at the arrow labeled "Taking Action from a Place of Meaning." This signifies that people in a social field "do what they do" together at any moment, because in the context of their social field those things make sense and have meaning for them.

Sometimes the team is working in routine patterns, and sometimes it is breaking those patterns in modes of learning. All of this is happening in flows of action and reflection by which the contextual resources and the social processes of the care team and its social field are continuously being made and re-made. All of this is in constant motion as the care team moves from existing routines into learning and back again – creating, maintaining, growing, collapsing, re-making and re-shaping the social field and all that the social field contains and makes possible.

If something new is tried, but the new ways don't make sense or matter, people will push them away. But if the new ways can be tried for a while longer, what makes sense and has meaning for people may evolve. So, an insight from this is to anchor anything new in established routines that make sense and matter to people, and to go slowly enough that the new ways will have time to change the context enough to take hold.

As shifts happen in what makes sense and has meaning in the care context, these shifts will be reflected and manifested in what people do together, in the social processes of the care team, and in the contextual resources of the social field.

It is interesting to ask how change happens in this model. The simple answer is: People act from what makes sense and has meaning for them. New ways of doing things gain a foothold and become established when the new ways make sense and have meaning for people. This is complex, because what people are doing together, what makes sense to them, and what has meaning to them can all be changing at once, reflexively, through their ongoing interactions, reflections, and conversations.

This insight that social fields are always in motion, constantly shaping and being shaped by ongoing interactions and conversations, is one of the most important contributions of the Social Field Model. Rather than viewing health care culture as resistant to change, something that must be "unfrozen" before change can happen, it is hopeful and useful to realize that social fields are dynamic, evolving contexts filled with potential.

Ongoing and full of potential

What is exciting about this understanding is that since social fields are always in motion, they are continuously open to change. One of the most interesting things to recognize from these insights is that social fields, and the resources carried in them, are created over time by people doing things together.

Like a river flowing, a social field has an apparent form and stability. However, if the shaping factors change in some way, like a river the social field will change too. This nature of social fields carries with it the promise of many possibilities beyond what presently exists. Part of the tension and aliveness of any team is because these things are always in motion. This understanding of social fields is exciting because it carries a lot of promise for collaborative care. We have found that the potential for achieving exceptional collaborative care can be counted on in every clinical unit we have studied and worked with. The building blocks are always present. New choices can be made, new routines can be started, and collaborative care can be created.

Summary: Social Field Model of Collaborative Care

The Social Field Model is based on principles of social construction which recognizes that people make sense and find meaning through conversations and interactions. The model, therefore, focuses on conversations and interactions in the care environment, and the conditions under which these occur.

The model seeks to implement collaborative care by intentionally establishing conditions in the care environment that are conducive to the emergence of collaborative ways of relating through new sense making and meaning making conversations.

The model points to conversations and interactions among care team members, patients, and family members as the way that collaborative social fields are built. Relational infrastructure sets the stage, and conversations and interactions enabled by relational infrastructure create and maintain collaborative social fields rich with contextual resources.

Relational infrastructure includes organizational practices that provide for consistent team interactions, reflective team meetings, collaborative rounds that include all professions with patients and families together, interprofessional leadership that emphasizes respectful, open communication and creates trust and psychological safety, and an infrastructure for learning and ongoing system improvement to achieve reliability and resilience.

The model views collaborative care as an emergent phenomenon that is likely to arise among health professionals, patients, and family members if these people are able to work together in a care environment that fosters, supports, and sustains collaborative ways of relating. These interactions establish and maintain a collaborative social field rich with contextual resources that the care team can draw from in its work together.

EPILOGUE

Mystery in going on

Very often when trying to help people who are navigating life and death, we reach places we've never been before.

Sometimes in those moments, nothing we have ever done before or experienced or figured out is able to help us understand what to do next. There is mystery in these moments, deep mystery. We want so much to do the right thing, and we have no way of knowing what that right thing might be.

Every human being faces these moments, and so does every collaborative care team. What can we say here that might help, in these moments of deepest mystery and loss of knowing? There are a handful of surprisingly simple guides. As collaborative care teams we are privileged to be present at these moments. There are so many levels.

The awe never goes away. In health care most of us remember so clearly how terrifying it was at first to come face to face with talking about death. Death itself was not terrifying. It was and remains full of mystery, but it has never been terrifying.

The terror, though, rests at the boundary of death and life – in the connections of love between people. In our lives in health care we have to tell many people horrible things that can have the effect of ripping apart the bonds of the connection that are at the center of human life.

There's no possible way this can be done well.

The terror of walking into that room, of looking into those faces, the feeling of pounding hearts and the holding of breaths, the knowing before knowing that waits in the room somehow before you even enter – all of these experiences and those that come next…

The anguished sounds that have no words, the sobs and tears, the rhythmic rocking, the comforting touch that cannot be felt, the helplessness and hopelessness and the anger and the determined disbelief giving way to a collapse that can never totally be made whole again...

And then the next waves, as others circle and hold, and feeling begins to return, and strength begins to flow from the most unexpected places – and gradually a kind of normalcy begins to regain a foothold, and questions can again be asked and answered, and plans, even the simplest of plans, can somehow again start to be made...

And in another room sheets are being changed, blood is being wiped from the floor, bloodstains are being covered, nose and mouth and hands are being washed and positioned, lights are being lowered, all with a reverence yet an efficiency that is also a mystery. And later the room is empty and the hallway is empty and the waiting room is empty. And, with the mystery, in empty spaces filled with the mystery, we go on.

It may be much smaller than this.

It may be simply sitting down as one person with another the night before surgery to talk about risks. Or maybe it is a simple question, "My son lives out of state. He's very busy at work this time of year. He wants to know if he should come. What should I tell him?"

In each of these moments there's never a right answer, a right thing to say, a right way to say it. The fascinating thing is – it doesn't matter, really, what is done. What matters is to take this big and impossible and terrifying thing and to make it as small as possible. Small, and authentic.

Recognizing that nothing can be said, yet... authentic presence, patient presence, caring presence, simply being with another for whatever time is necessary, is often the only and most precious gift that can be given.

We are changed forever by these moments. In ways small and large, the experiences of moving together through these times of mystery shape us, inform us, deplete us, and restore us. Often, we do not even know that they are coming. Often we do not even know of the surprising strengths that these moments reveal when called upon, and the bedrock that we touch when all else is suddenly gone.

The only thing that we know for sure about these moments is the importance of taking time. Time makes the terror small. It looks the terror calmly in the eye and says, "We are here." "We will wait. We will be patient. And in the end, we will forgive and heal, and we will go on."

And then there are the other days – when the mystery is equally present but the outcome is very different. Blood pressure stabilizes. Bleeding stops. Oxygen levels improve. A patient wakes up who had little hope for recovery.

Our team had one of those days recently. A young mother with four children is alive today by some miracle. In part, it was a human miracle.

Diane helped by opening the patient's chest with no chest instruments, somehow getting the sternum open with a pair of heavy scissors so she could get her hand on the one inch hole in the superior vena cava. Shawn and Amy helped by pumping in blood, fresh frozen plasma, platelets and cryoprecipitate, keeping up with half a blood volume lost, while managing pressors and ventilation.

Marilyn and Teresa and Kim helped by turning the chaos of an unexpected resuscitation into the controlled intensity of a smoothly functioning cardiac operating room. Paul and Don helped by establishing a stable surgical field and sewing the hole closed; Tredessa helped with the heart lung machine.

Christina and Nathalie helped by exceptional nursing care in the ICU. Cherise helped by supporting the family through a long day and night. And many others helped in ways we may never even know.

Later, driving home in the morning sun, this thought comes:

"If we do nothing else – ever – than give those children back their mom…that is enough."

A week later the memories are:

The first response to her name; the first glances at her children; her first written notes; the words of her daughter, "She is our same old Mom!" The breathing tube coming out; the comforting hand of her best friend; the attentive patience of her husband, their shared look and a whispered, "I love you. Don't you ever leave me"…

The first chip of ice; the drawings on the wall from her children; the first time to the chair; the tubes coming out; the first bites of applesauce; the transfer out of the ICU; the reassurance; the smiles; and the happiness of a homecoming.

We do this for that.

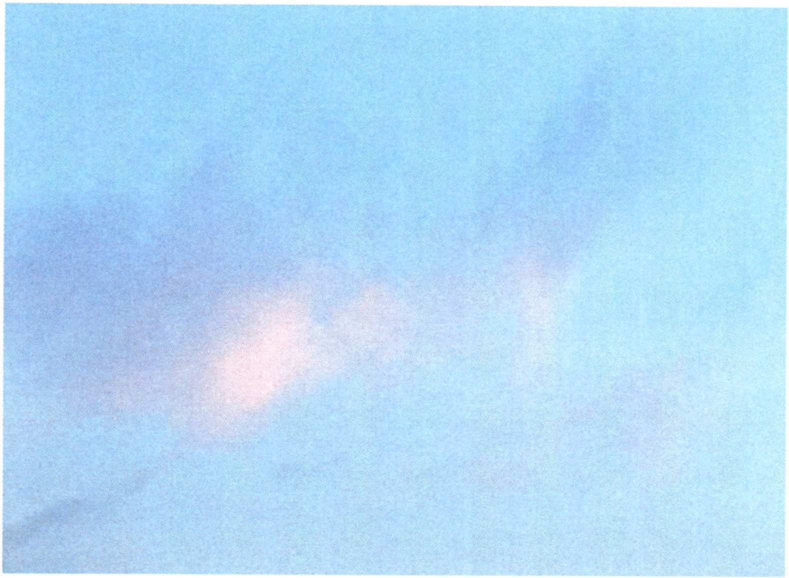

HISTORY OF THIS WORK

The *Field Guide to Collaborative Care* contains the ideas, work, and contributions of many people including patients, family members, care team members, and researchers from many care environments. It is a guide and reference developed by those who share a commitment to exploring how health care can become even better through collaboration across professions, with active engagement of patients and families.

As authors, we are privileged to give these ideas this particular form and structure. However, what is presented here extends far beyond us. We recognize with gratitude the pioneering work of Jeff Brown, Addie Camelio, Anne Nason, Elise Kendall and others at Concord Hospital, Concord, NH, who helped develop this approach to care. We also thank research colleagues Cindy Dominguez, Lorri Zipperer, Olga Gurevich, Gerry Stahl, Alan Zemel, and Wes Shumar, all members of the original MGH "Way Cool X-Team." We are grateful for other friends and colleagues whose support has been essential to the development of the Field Guide, including Sheila McNamee, Sara Singer, Jody Gittell, Margie Godfrey, Baron Hamman and Gene Beyt, who helped co-found the Collaborative Care Alliance.

The *Field Guide to Collaborative Care* is a story of perseverance, insights, joys, sorrows, and the unexpected. It is a record of what we have learned together with patients, families, and colleagues – successes achieved, mistakes made, and our best understanding of what matters, and why. It is a work in progress that is far from complete. This section describes its beginnings and history.

The *Field Guide to Collaborative Care* had its origin in the work of care team members, patients, and family members of the cardiac surgery program at Concord Hospital (Concord, New Hampshire), who together developed the Concord Collaborative Care Model in 1999-2003.

The Concord Collaborative Care Model was based on principles of Human Factors Science, Safety Science, High Reliability Organization Theory, and Patient and Family Centered Care. These principles were "woven into the fabric" of the communications processes and daily interactions that occurred among clinical care team members, patients, and family members.

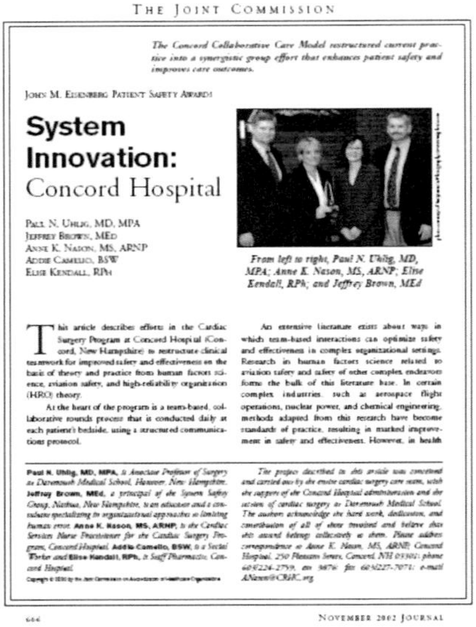

THE JOINT COMMISSION

The Concord Collaborative Care Model restructured current practice into a synergistic group effort that enhances patient safety and improves care outcomes.

JOHN M. EISENBERG PATIENT SAFETY AWARDS

System Innovation:
Concord Hospital

PAUL N. UHLIG, MD, MPA
JEFFREY BROWN, MED
ANNE K. NASON, MS, ARNP
ADDIE CAMELIO, BSW
ELISE KENDALL, RPH

From left to right, Paul N. Uhlig, MD, MPA; Anne K. Nason, MS, ARNP; Elise Kendall, RPh; and Jeffrey Brown, MEd

This article describes efforts in the Cardiac Surgery Program at Concord Hospital (Concord, New Hampshire) to restructure clinical teamwork for improved safety and effectiveness on the basis of theory and practice from human factors science, aviation safety, and high-reliability organization (HRO) theory.

At the heart of the program is a team-based, collaborative rounds process that is conducted daily at each patient's bedside, using a structured communications protocol.

An extensive literature exists about ways in which team-based interactions can optimize safety and effectiveness in complex organizational settings. Research in human factors science related to aviation safety and safety of other complex endeavors forms the bulk of this literature base. In certain complex industries such as aerospace flight operations, nuclear power, and chemical engineering, methods adapted from this research have become standards of practice, resulting in marked improvement in safety and effectiveness. However, in health

666 NOVEMBER 2002 JOURNAL

The Concord Hospital team, together with safety scientist and advisor Jeffrey Brown, received the 2002 John M. Eisenberg Patient Safety Award in System Innovation from the Joint Commission and National Quality Forum.

Implementation of the Collaborative Care Model at Concord Hospital was associated with notable improvements in care outcomes, patient satisfaction, and quality of work life.

The *Field Guide to Collaborative Care* is written from experiences during this initial work, and additional field experiences with collaborative care teams at the University of

Cincinnati from 2005-2006; in Wichita, Kansas, from 2007-2012; and in Salina, Kansas, from 2012-2015.

The work is also informed by research studies of collaborative care by a core group of collaborating investigators. The first was a study of the Collaborative Care Model funded by the Information Systems Research Council of Partners Health Care/ Massachusetts General Hospital, Boston, Massachusetts.

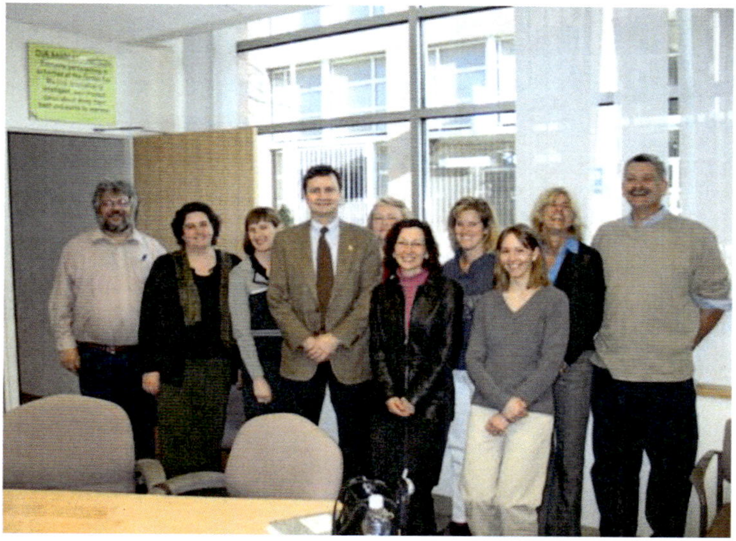

Photo: Preparing for a collaborative rounds simulation, Center for Medical Simulation, Cambridge, Massachusetts, 2004

Observations, interviews, video analysis and ethnography were used to study the patterns of interaction of clinical team members, patients, and family members across a spectrum of clinical settings during clinical care and in simulation scenarios.

Goals of the study were to characterize how collaborative practice differs from traditional practice; understand why the

Collaborative Care Model works and how it improves care; predict its stability in different organizational cultures; develop methods to implement and support the Collaborative Care Model in various clinical settings; and consider ways that innovative information systems could be designed to support collaborative practice.

Members of this research team included Paul Uhlig, Jeff Brown, Addie Camelio, Cindy Dominguez, Olga Gurevich, Wes Shumar, Gerry Stahl, Alan Zemel, and Lorri Zipperer. Important contributions were made by Elise Kendall, Kate Gillen, Anita Tucker, Hank Grinvalsky, and Katherine Klein. Support and advocacy for this project were provided by Nathaniel Sims, Jeffrey Cooper, Dan Raemer, Andrew Warshaw, and John Glaser.

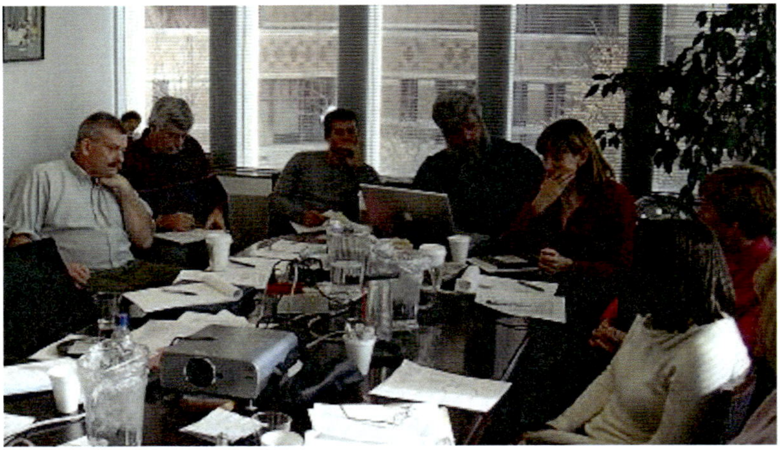

Photo: Research Team Meeting, Cincinnati, Ohio, 2006

In 2006, Sara Singer, then co-director of the Stanford Patient Safety Consortium, asked whether the Concord Collaborative Care Model could be developed into a guide to be offered as a patient safety culture intervention for participating hospitals. A group of initial authors, including Paul Uhlig, Ellen Raboin, Jeff Brown, Katherine Klein, Sara Singer and Alyson

Falwell, began collaborating to create such a resource. After nine years the *Field Guide to Collaborative Care* is the culmination of this writing effort.

A second major study informing the *Field Guide to Collaborative Care* is field research for the PhD dissertation research of Ellen Raboin, conducted in 2009. Ellen studied the development of collaborative practice among a care team on a medical surgical unit in an acute care hospital.

Ellen focused attention on the role of conversations in reconstructing relationships between the multiple professionals of the collaborative care team, patients and family members, private physicians, and the hospital organization. Her research was undertaken from a social construction orientation, and the ideas developed in this research have informed the theories underlying the Social Field Model of Collaborative Care.

The third study informing the Field Guide was funded by the Wichita Center for Graduate Medical Education and the Kansas Biosciences Authority, under the auspices of the Kansas University School of Medicine-Wichita. Field work was conducted in 2010-2012, and analysis and writing are being completed.

This study is a mixed methods participatory research study actively engaging care team members, patients, and family members as co-researchers, studying the development of collaborative care on the cardiac surgery service at a community hospital.

Members of the Kansas research team included Paul Uhlig, Ellen Raboin, Jeff Brown, Cindy Dominguez, Lorri Zipperer, Karen Kramer, Diana Lippoldt, and Joann Paul. Additional contributions were made by Eli Brumfield. Participating care team members, patients, and family members included Bob Baker, Jim

Catt, Paula Cook, Diane Dorsch, Carolyn Earnest, Marilyn Ehrhart, Debbie Fox, John Irving, Charissa Jochems, Dan Jordan, Kent Jossie, Carolyn Kitchens, Bridgette Kram, Lora Lagree, Gary Miller, Marcy Moore, Vanessa Porter, Jane Siebert, Joyce Wooding and Jim Yock. The support of David Grainger, Robert McKay, Doug Bradham, H. David Wilson, Kathy Neely, and Francie Ekengren helped to make this study possible.

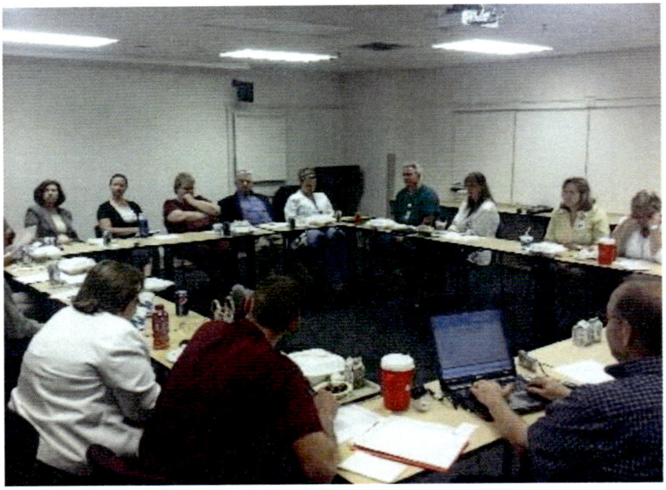

Photo: Participatory collaborative care research, Wichita, Kansas, 2011

We are also indebted to many other clinical teams, patients and family members, and clinical leaders from many sites, especially from University Hospital, Cincinnati, Ohio; North Shore Medical Center in Salem, Massachusetts; Salina Regional Health Center in Salina, Kansas; University Hospital and University of Texas Health Science Center at San Antonio, Texas; and Magee Women's Hospital in Pittsburgh, Pennsylvania, whose efforts to improve care, enhance reliability and resilience, and increase patient and family engagement have been instrumental in refining the recommendations in the *Field Guide to Collaborative Care*.

In closing, it is important to recognize that this work is part of a broader movement. In the past two decades, remarkable advances have been made in understanding patient safety and health care teamwork. You will see insights and influences in this book from the researchers and practitioners listed below, in and out of health care. We have had the privilege of sharing ideas with many of these pioneering researchers as colleagues and friends. We admire and honor them for their gifts and contributions.

Safety Science	James Reason, Charles Vincent
Safety in Health Care	Lucian Leape, Jeff Cooper, Julie Morath
Safety Culture and Climate	Bryan Sexton, Robert Helmreich
Patient/Family Centered Care	Susan Edgman-Levitan, Bev Johnson
Relationship Centered Care	Anthony Suchman, Dana Safran
Distributed Cognition	Edwin Hutchins
High Reliability Organizations	Karlene Roberts, Kathleen Sutcliff, Karl Weick, Tim Vogus, Sara Singer
Clinical Microsystems	Marjorie Godfrey, Gene Nelson, Paul Batalden, Julie Mohr
Relational Social Construction	Sheila McNamee, Ken Gergen
Appreciative Inquiry	David Cooperrider
Making Social Worlds	Barnett Pearce
Complexity Science	Ralph Stacey, Paul Plsek, Curt Lindberg
Transformative Group Process	Peter Block
Organizational Culture	Edgar Schein
Structuration Theory	Anthony Giddens
Relational Coordination	Jody Gittell
Front Line Problem Solving	Anita Tucker
Team Learning	Amy Edmondson
Positive Deviance	Jerry and Monique Sternin, Jon Lloyd
Collaborative Learning	Gerry Stahl, Wes Shumar, Alan Zemel
Resilience Engineering	David Woods, Erik Hollnagel, Sidney Dekker
Simulation	Dan Raemer, Jeff Cooper, David Gaba
Unit based Safety Interventions	Peter Pronovost, Christine Goeschel
Interprofessional Education	John Gilbert, Barbara Brandt, Amy Blue
Naturalistic Decision Making	Gary Klein, Chris Nemeth
Teamwork and Team Training	Eduardo Salas, Robert Simon
Non-Technical Teamwork Skills	Rona Flin, Luci McDonald, Stephen Yule

GLOSSARY and INDEX OF KEY IDEAS

Action-Reflection Learning Systems (165-171)

A process and an infrastructure that connects doing with learning to produce reliability and resilience. Key components are collective patterns for action, structural opportunities for collective reflection/change, and trust.

Collaborative Care (21-31)

Exceptional health care in which patients, family members, and other care team members are able to consistently co-create care that is meaningful, high quality, efficient, safe, reliable, resilient, and exquisitely responsive to the hopes, needs, goals, and purposes of everyone involved.

Contextual Resources (234-238)

Special capabilities of collaborative teams that arise over time in a particular social field as the team works and learns together. Once contextual resources are established, a team is able to use these resources in its day to day activities. Contextual resources in social fields make reliability and resilience possible.

Curve 1 and Curve 2 Health Care (11-13)

Based on ideas of Ian Morrison and Martin Merry, Curve 1 is the current era of health care, and Curve 2 is a transformational new paradigm coming into existence through pioneering models such as collaborative care.

Knowing Smile (225-227)

A look between people that signifies much more than is obvious. With a quick glance an entire past history of information, memory, emotions, and shared experiences can flow between people without a word being spoken.

Natural Work Cluster (68-76)

A set of roles and resources that consistently come together in response to a pattern of need. Aligning organizational boundaries with natural work clusters is a foundational organizing principle in the Social Field Model.

Preconditions (55-58)

Certain structural and social attributes of the care environment that support the emergence of collaborative care and can be intentionally strengthened. The Social Field Model focuses on strengthening preconditions as the primary approach for implementing collaborative care.

Relational Infrastructure (243-245)

Anything in the care environment that supports the development of productive working relationships among care team members, patients, and family members.

Reliability (186-197)

The ability of a care team to consistently do whatever it intends to do, across a wide set of possible circumstances.

Resilience (186-197)

The ability of a care team to productively adapt and respond when encountering the unexpected.

Social Construction (239-243)

A field of scholarship that focuses on what is made or "socially constructed" as people interact and converse. The Social Field Model of Collaborative Care is based on concepts and principles of social construction.

Social Field (225-233)

A living collective intelligence of accumulated experiences, memories and connections that grows over time among members of a team who are able to work together regularly and reflect together about their interactions. The abilities of exceptional teams develop and are applied in social fields.

Social Field Model of Collaborative Care (245-253)

A theoretical and practical model based in principles of social construction that is useful for understanding and guiding the implementation of collaborative care and for understanding and achieving reliability and resilience.

Team-Level Tacit Knowledge (230-233)

Team-level knowledge of how to do things in ways that are learned from experience and can't be written down. Social fields carry extensive team-level tacit knowledge.

Type 1 and Type 2 Problem Solving (181-182)

Based on the work of Anita Tucker, first order or Type 1 problem solving is doing something that solves an immediate concern but doesn't change the underlying root condition. Second order or Type 2 problem solving addresses the concern at a root level. Achieving reliability requires team-level Type 2 problem-solving capability.

COLLABORATIVE CARE LEARNING NETWORK

If you would like to learn more about collaborative care and the Social Field Model of Collaborative Care, we encourage you to participate in the **Collaborative Care Learning Network.**

You can find out more about the **Collaborative Care Learning Network** and download the latest versions of the **Collaborative Care Toolkit**, including the Collaborative Care TEAMFINDER, Collaborative Care Activation Inventory (CCAI), and the Collaborative Care Resource Inventory (CCRI), on the **Collaborative Care Alliance website** at www.cca-home.org.

We invite and welcome you!

ABOUT THE AUTHORS

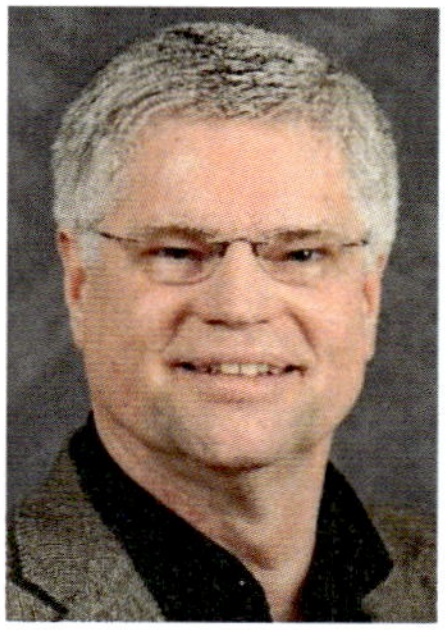

Paul Uhlig, MD, MPA, is a cardiothoracic surgeon. Paul's practice and research explores how health care can become safer, more meaningful, more effective, and more efficient through collaborative care with active engagement of patients and families. He has given invited presentations about collaborative care across the US and internationally, including the Royal College of Surgeons of Edinburgh where he was honored with a King James IV Professorship. Paul trained as a physician at the University of Kansas; as a surgeon at the Massachusetts General Hospital and Indiana University; as a researcher at the University of California San Francisco; and received a Mid-Career Master of Public Administration degree from Harvard University.

Ellen Raboin, PhD, MSOD, MBA, is a researcher and consultant with special expertise in social construction and the Coordinated Management of Meaning. Ellen's work makes human systems visible, connects people, and explores the meaning of health and healing in human systems in support of health care transformation. She holds a Doctorate in Human and Organization Systems from Fielding Graduate University, a Masters in Organization Development from Pepperdine University, a MBA from Cal State, a BS in Chemical Engineering from Georgia Institute of Technology, and BA from Berry College. Ellen is President of the Board of Directors of the Ronald McDonald House of San Francisco.

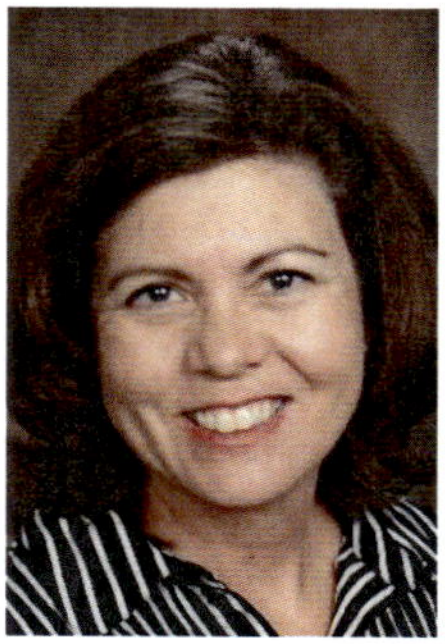